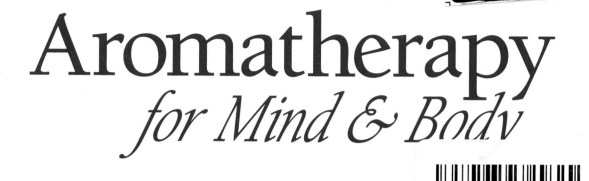

Aromatherapy
for Mind & Body

David Schiller & Carol Schiller

Sterling Publishing Co., Inc.
New York

Before using any of the formulas, please read carefully Chapter 3, "The Safety and Handling of Oils." The safe and proper use of the oils is the sole responsibility of the reader. The authors and publisher assume no responsibility or liability for anyone's misuse, carelessness, allergic reactions, skin sensitivity, or any other conditions arising directly or indirectly from the use of this book. This book is not intended to replace the services of a physician.

ACKNOWLEDGMENTS

We would like to thank these special people who contributed their valuable efforts towards the production of this book: Jeffrey Schiller; Rochelle Schiller; Roslyn Blumenthal; the librarians and staff at the Maricopa Public Library in Arizona, Connie Delpier and Marrian Malone; and all the wonderful people at Sterling Publishing Company, especially Sheila Anne Barry, acquisitions director; John Woodside, editorial director; Hannah Steinmetz, editor; and Charles Nurnberg, executive vice president.

Library of Congress Cataloging-in-Publication Data

Schiller, David.
    Aromatherapy for mind & body / David Schiller & Carol Schiller.
        p.   cm.
    Includes index.
    ISBN 0-8069-4244-4
    1. Aromatherapy.   I. Schiller, Carol.   II. Title.
    RM666.A68S353   1996
    615´.321—dc20   95-46738
                                                                                    CIP

1   3   5   7   9   10   8   6   4   2

Published by Sterling Publishing Company, Inc.
387 Park Avenue South, New York, N.Y. 10016
© 1996 by Carol Schiller and David Schiller
Distributed in Canada by Sterling Publishing
c/o Canadian Manda Group, One Atlantic Avenue, Suite 105
Toronto, Ontario, Canada M6K 3E7
Distributed in Great Britain and Europe by Cassell PLC
Wellington House, 125 Strand, London WC2R 0BB, England
Distributed in Australia by Capricorn Link (Australia) Pty Ltd.
P.O. Box 6651, Baulkham Hills, Business Centre, NSW 2153, Australia
Manufactured in the United States of America
All rights reserved

Sterling ISBN 0-8069-4244-4

As a shining light allows us vision in the midst of darkness—a precious essence vaporizing its fragrantly scented molecules awakens the senses, kindles the spirit and enhances our overall well-being by bringing the life-giving force of nature into our life.
—David Schiller and Carol Schiller

CONTENTS

THE ESSENCE OF NATURE

❂ ❂ ❂

THE SUBLIME FRAGRANCES emitted by aromatic trees and plants in bloom, ushering in feelings of excitement and joy as the beautiful season of spring arrives. The rejuvenating clean, fresh air of a pine and spruce forest after a rain shower. The strikingly brilliant colors of autumn leaves as they contrast against the clear blue sky. The hypnotic scents of jasmine and tuberose flowers perfuming the summer midnight air, setting a romantic ambience for lovers.

These are some of the marvelous wonders of nature.

Throughout history, various cultures have respected nature to the degree of worship. Pantheism is the belief that God is present in all elements of the natural world. The followers of Shintoism, the oldest surviving religion in Japan, worship gods that are believed to be the basic force of mountains, trees, rocks, rivers, and other parts of nature. The Jain religion in India considers all life sacred and forbids the uprooting of trees, removal of unripe fruits, tearing of leaves, and the pulling off of flowers.

The ancient Greeks held sacred the olive and cypress trees. The Hindus believe trees like the pipal tree to be holy and that worshiping and eating the leaves of the neem tree prevent illness. The Hindus and Muslims revere the sandalwood tree and use its incense in various religious ceremonies and funeral services. Ojibway Indians of North America are reluctant to fell a tree for fear of causing it pain. The coconut palm is sanctified in New Guinea. Its wood, bark, leaves, and fruit provide food, shelter, clothing, utensils, and objects used for religious ceremonies.

During the past century, however, people drifted away and became estranged from the natural environment. The use of toxic chemicals to produce fibres, consumer products, and on food crops vastly proliferated. In addition, great numbers of people left small towns and farm life in favor of the big city.

The benefits of urban living appeared very appealing: more lucrative employment opportunities and thus potential for a higher standard of living, greater opportunities to socialize, and easy access to a larger variety of foods, goods, places to visit, and events to attend.

In the city the saying is, "Time is money." Everyone always seems to be in a hurry. The sounds of nature are overtaken by screeching brakes as vehicles stop at traffic lights, loud emergency sirens, blasting automobile horns, jackhammers, and construction noise.

Besides the noise, in many areas the polluted air can be seen as well as smelled.

As ailments caused by stress and pollution mount each year, larger numbers of people are increasingly taking action to help themselves. Shiatsu, therapeutic massage, yoga, deep relaxation exercises, visualization, meditation, and aromatherapy are among the measures practiced that have grown the fastest in recent years, as people try to reverse the deleterious effects of urban living.

Aromatherapy is the use of pure essential oils, which are the essences extracted from trees, shrubs, flowers, herbs, and grasses. These precious oils can be used in myriad ways—to enjoy a candlelight dinner in a delightful, aromatic setting; to scent and purify the air to improve the indoor environment; to enhance a therapeutic or loving massage; to surrender stress, to revitalize hair and skin and reduce cellulite for a shapely body. Prepare your own deodorants, mouthwashes, bath oils, moisturizers for chapped lips, and facial cremes to keep your skin young and beautiful.

The formulas for yoga can help you become more limber by making it easier to stretch your muscles and ligaments. If you are stressed and wish to relax in a sauna or steam bath, you'll enjoy the special sauna/steam room stress-reducing mist sprays. The jock- and jane-itch powders can offer great relief. If you shave, you'll find a choice of pre-shave powders and shaving cremes. When a snorer in the house keeps you awake, the stop-snoring spray mist formulas will be right there to assist you.

Perhaps you'd like to achieve a goal you haven't been able to accomplish before. The oils can help you enter into a relaxed state to improve your visualization skills and gain more insight from your intuition. You will also find the introspection, appreciation, improvement, loving yourself, and meditation exercises very helpful. The mental concentration formulas can help improve your ability to focus on problem solving using the faculties of logic and reason.

So, attain higher achievements, create more happiness and joy within yourself, enrich your relationships, become a good role model for others to follow, pursue a higher purpose, make a difference, and put more meaning into your life.

Appreciate the natural surroundings as often as you can: Remove your shoes, walk barefoot on a lawn or in the countryside and feel the soft green grass caressing the bottoms of your feet. Grow your own vegetable garden and enjoy a salad from the freshly gathered vegetables; spend time on an unspoiled mountain with pleasing scenery around you; watch a beautiful sunset; bathe in a lake of pristine waters; brush delicate silky flower petals gently against your skin and relish their delightful fragrance.

When you return home from the wonderful experiences of nature, use the essential oils as an extension of the natural atmosphere. Indulge in as many formulas as you wish. Don't deny yourself the pleasure, take advantage of the benefits awaiting you, and make every day a special one from now on!

CHAPTER 1

AROMA COMMUNICATION

✿ ✿ ✿

IN NATURE, SCENT plays a major role in the survival of a species. Flowers that aren't pollinated by airborne pollen produce a scent to attract insects and animals. For pollination, these plants enter into a symbiotic relationship with other living beings.

Animals use aroma communication for mating and to mark their territories. Fish use scent to alert other fish to danger. Aroma communication is not as profoundly used by humans, but still we are greatly affected.

The process of communication through scent is a highly fascinating aspect of the natural world.

INSECTS

The female bolas spider spins a strand at the end of which is a sticky substance containing a chemical that replicates the sexual scent of a female moth. The male moth is attracted by the smell and when he approaches, he becomes stuck on the lure and is caught by the spider.

Ants mark their trail on the ground depositing a small amount of pheromone substance for the other ants to follow. This signal is vital to communicate the discovery of a new supply of food. It has been calculated that one milligram of this pheromone substance could lead a column of ants three times around the earth!

The male Chinese emperor moth can detect the female pheromone from over six miles away. The male silkworm moth has the ability to sense a smell a distance of two miles away.

ANIMALS

The male mink lets off a musky vapor from glands beside his anus. To the human, this musky odor is unpleasant, but in the female mink it creates a feeling of ecstasy leading to mating.

Rabbits, squirrels, and hares use urine in courtship. A courting male hare entices a female by taking great leaps. While he is airborne he showers the female with urine. It is presumed by this act that the female smells the male hormones in the urine and the sexual response follows.

The sow attracts the boar and allows him to mount her after becoming excited by seeing him, hearing the sounds he makes, and especially smelling his musky breath.

The female hamster makes a trail of vaginal secretions by dragging her hind legs along the ground. When the male senses the smell, he responds by following it to the female, who anxiously awaits him. A male hamster who is unable to smell will fail to respond to a female.

The male reindeer leaves secretion deposits from a gland between its toes. The scent discourages other males from entering into this marked territory.

HUMANS

Studies show that during the first two months of life, infants increasingly display a preference for the smell of their mother's breast over that of other women. The reverse is also true. In one study, the mothers were blindfolded and presented a choice of three babies. Sixty-one percent of the mothers correctly selected their own baby.

Menstrual cycles of women who live together become synchronized over a period of several months. There is speculation that this is due to each woman being exposed to the other woman's perspiration smell, and adapting to the other woman's cycle.

In a study, perspiration collected from men's underarms was swabbed three times a week on the upper lips of women whose cycles were irregular. After three months, all the women's cycles were regulated to 29.5 days.

Studies have also shown that women who are around men have more regulated cycles and men who are around women have more rapid hair growth.

PLANTS

The orchid belongs to a large family of about 20,000 plants having beautiful flowers and assorted colors. The plants range in size from ¼ inch (0.6 cm) to large vines 100 feet (30 m) long. The orchids have adapted their color, image, and scent to suit their individual needs in order to survive.

Part of the flower of hammer orchid, of the *Drakaea* species in Australia, resembles a female wasp. The male wasps emerge about two weeks earlier than the females and the orchids take full advantage of the time difference. The flowers open and emit a scent similar to the female wasps just during the time period the male wasps appear. Driven by the mating instinct, the male wasp lands on the flower and attempts to mate with it. His actions trigger a lever in the lobe of the flower that throws him into the flower head-first. As the wasp struggles to escape, the pollen sacks become stuck to his back. Afterwards when the wasp visits another flower of the same species, the process is repeated and the pollen from the previous flower is transferred to the new one for pollination.

The Mediterranean *Ophrys* species orchid secretes a chemical scent similar to the pheromone of a female wasp. This scent lures the male wasp to the flower. During the pseudocopulation the pollen mass sticks to the male wasp, which then transports it to the stigma of the next flower of the same species.

In the tropics, orchids of the genus

Trichoceros mimic female flies and are pollinated by sexually aroused males.

The lady's slipper orchid (*Cypripedium cacceolus)* produces a nectar-like scent. It is so slippery that a visiting bee slides down into the flower and can only exit by squeezing through a narrow path that causes the bee to become laden with pollen.

In 1982, biologists Drs. Gordon Orians and David Rhoades conducted a research project for the University of Washington. They deliberately placed caterpillars and webworms on willow and alder trees to determine how the trees would respond to these predators. Within hours of the infestation, the chemical composition of the leaves began to change. Chemicals known as terpenes and tannins were produced and the protein content became altered. This caused the leaves to become indigestible. The insects starved and began to die.

However, the most remarkable discovery was that nearby trees, which were not under attack by the insects, began to produce the same defenses—even though these trees were at a distance from one another and there wasn't any physical contact between their root systems or branches.

The scientists concluded that the infested trees communicated with the other trees by releasing airborne chemicals known as aroma molecules.

CHAPTER 2

HOW TO USE AROMATHERAPY

✵ ✵ ✵

ESSENTIAL OILS ARE FRAGRANT oily components extracted from petals of flowers, leaves, roots, seeds, fruits, woods, grasses, and resins. Some plants yield oil from only one part, while others contain oil in several parts. Orange trees yield oil from the flowers, twigs, leaves, and rind of the fruit. The leaves, buds, and stems from the clove tree contain oil, while only the fruits from the tree of litsea cubeba are used to produce an essential oil.

The quality and quantity of essential oil produced depends on various factors: location where the plant is grown, altitude, moisture, climate, condition of soil, and even the season or time of day or night the plant material is harvested. The extraction process also plays a key role in the quality of an oil. Steam distillation, carbon dioxide extraction, and cold-pressed oils are preferable, while solvent-extracted oil should be avoided, since harmful chemicals are used in the extraction process.

Essential oils, sometimes referred to as ethereal substances, are certainly more than just nice smelling. The oils can be used simply and effectively to scent and beautify the body, create a wonderful environment, and help promote inner peace and thus a happier mental state.

Here are methods that can be employed to use these marvelous aromatic oils:

APPLICATION

In this self-application method, apply the oil on the skin, rubbing it in until it is fully absorbed. Application is used when a massage is not absolutely necessary.

AROMA LAMPS

An aroma lamp has a small container that is heated after water and essential oils are added. When the water becomes hot the aromatic vapors are dispersed into the air.

BATHS

Throughout history, public baths served as social centers. In some cultures, bathing is an important part of daily life for cleansing. Baths can be very beneficial to health, and they serve as a delightful therapeutic measure to relax and calm or invigorate and refresh the body. An aromatherapy bath can be so pleasurable it can become an anticipated and planned-for event.

Directions: Close the bathroom door and window to keep the essential oil vapors from escaping. Play soft music you enjoy listening to. Fill the bathtub with water as warm as you like. Then mix the essential oils with the carrier oil and add the blend to the bathwater. Swirl the water to distribute the oils evenly throughout the tub. Enter the bath immediately.

BODY POWDERS

Body powders are used to scent, deodorize, and disinfect the skin.

Directions: Measure the amount of cornstarch needed and pour into a small widemouthed glass jar, then add the essential oils. Mix the ingredients thoroughly. Allow the powder to sit for a day before use.

CREMES

Cremes are very useful aromatherapy products. They are easy to apply, readily absorb into the skin, and have a smooth texture. Natural vegetable butter is used as a medium in the cremes in this book.

Directions: Place the indicated amount of vegetable butter in a wide-mouthed glass jar, put the jar into a small pot of water, and heat. When the butter is melted add the carrier oil, mix well, and remove from the heat. As the mixture cools, add the essential oils and stir well.

DIFFUSORS

Diffusors disperse a mist of microparticles of essential oil, which creates an aromatic atmosphere indoors. Different types of diffusors are available on the market. Choose a smaller or larger unit, depending on the size of the area to be fragranced. The formulas given for diffusor use are in percentages rather than drops due to the different types of units. In one type, essential oils are added to a pad that is vaporized by an electric fan. A second type has a small glass bottle that essential oils are placed into. The oil is then propelled into a nebulizer and vaporized into the air. A third type requires the essential oils to be placed on a pad and releases the vapors though a warming process.

FACIAL SAUNA

This method is used as a facial cleansing treatment and to open clogged pores and revitalize problem skin.

Directions: Heat a small pot of water and pour it into a bowl, then add the essential oils. Immediately drape a towel over your head to form a tent over the bowl. Close your eyes, and lean over towards the vapors for five to 10 minutes.

LIGHT BULB RINGS

Directions: Place the light bulb ring on top of a cool light bulb and drop the essential oils into the groove of the ring. When the light is turned on, the bulb is heated, dispersing the aromatic vapors into the air.

MASSAGE

An aromatherapy massage can provide a means of counteracting pressures of daily life. Only after receiving a massage do we realize how tight our muscles have been and the high amounts of tension stored in our body. Some people think of massage as a luxury and utilize it only in times of severe distress. But living under the strain of modern society, we should recognize massage as an extraordinarily beneficial measure for stressed individuals to receive on a regular basis.

For best results when giving or receiving a massage, please follow these guidelines:

- The room should be quiet, warm, and comfortable.
- Soft music can be played to promote relaxation.
- Mist a nice essential oil fragrance in the room before the treatment.
- Be in a calm state before giving the massage. Tension can be easily transferred from one person to another.
- Make sure your fingernails are short before giving a massage, to avoid scratching the recipient's skin.
- All jewelry should be removed.
- A firm cushion can be used if a massage table is unavailable. The recipient should be covered with a sheet or blanket for warmth.
- Choose the appropriate aromatherapy massage formula and place all oils nearby to avoid searching for them during the massage.
- Wash hands with warm/hot water before and after giving the massage.
- Wear comfortable clothing.
- Warm the carrier/base oil by placing the small container in warm water. Pour an ample amount into the palm of your hand, rub hands together, and apply the oil on the recipient's skin.

MIST SPRAYS

A convenient and effective way to disperse aromatic vapors into the air is through the use of a mist spray. As the aromas mature in the bottle, the fragrance improves and becomes more pleasant.

Directions: Fill a four ounce (120 ml) fine mist spray bottle with purified water and add the essential oils. Tighten the cap and shake well.

To use: Shake the bottle well. Sit comfortably in a chair, close your eyes, spray the mist approximately 10 times over your head (2–3 sprays at a time), and take slow, deep breaths, breathing the vapors deeply. Use indoors for the full benefit.

SAUNA/STEAM ROOM

Saunas and steam rooms are perhaps the greatest places to loosen the muscles, rid the body of impurities, and relieve stress. Mist sprays are especially useful to help the breathing passages, in addition to pleasurably scenting the air.

Directions: See instructions for mist sprays. When using, spray away from the face, with eyes closed, so vapors do not irritate the eyes.

STEAM INHALATION

This method is usually employed to open the breathing passages.

Directions: Heat a small pot of water and pour it into a bowl, then add the essential oils. Immediately drape a towel over your head, close your eyes, and lean over towards the vapors. Inhale deeply.

CHAPTER 3

THE SAFETY AND HANDLING OF OILS

✦ ✦ ✦

SAFETY

To ensure safe use of essential oils please adhere to the following:

• Essential oils are highly concentrated substances and should be diluted in a carrier oil before being applied to the skin. Some of the common carrier oils are almond (sweet), apricot kernel, avocado, borage, flaxseed, grape seed, hazelnut, jojoba, kukui nut, sesame, sunflower, walnut.

• Only pure essential oils and pure unrefined carrier oils should be used. Never purchase oils that are solvent extracted, synthetic, or refined. The refining process removes valuable nutrients, and chemical preservatives are added to extend the shelf life of the product.

• The oils of basil (sweet), bergamot, cinnamon leaf, clove, grapefruit, lemon, lemongrass, lime, mandarin, orange, pepper (black), peppermint, spearmint, and tangerine can irritate the skin, especially dry skin. If any skin irritation should occur as a result of the essential oils, immediately apply lavender oil neat or a carrier oil to the area. This will quickly soothe the skin.

• If a person is sensitive, the number of drops of essential oils in the massage and bath oil formulas can be reduced to make the formulas half-strength.

• When applying essential oils on the skin, using a spray mist, or taking a scented bath be careful not to get essential oil vapors into the eyes. If the oils have already irritated the eyes, flush with cool water.

• Care should be taken when using carrier and essential oils during pregnancy. Many of the oils have a stimulating effect on the uterus that can be very helpful at the appropriate time to facilitate childbirth. However, if those oils are used prior to the time of childbirth, they can bring on premature labor. Even certain common foods, spices, and vegetable oils—celery, carrots, parsley, basil, bay leaves, marjoram, and safflower oil, for example—can stimulate uterine contractions.

• Small amounts (2–3 drops at a time) of the following essential oils are safe during pregnancy: bergamot, coriander, cypress, frankincense, geranium, ginger, grapefruit, lavender, lemon, lime, mandarin, neroli, orange, patchouli, petitgrain, sandalwood, spearmint, tangerine, tea tree, and ylang-ylang. Sesame oil can be used as a carrier oil.

- If a person is highly allergic, a simple test can determine if there is any sensitivity to a particular oil. Rub a drop of carrier oil on the upper chest area, and in 12 hours check for redness or any other skin reaction. If the skin is clear, place one drop of an essential oil, diluted in 15 drops of the same carrier oil, and again rub on the upper chest area. If there is no skin reaction after 12 hours, both carrier and essential oil can be used.
- Do not consume alcohol, except a small glass of wine with a meal, in the time period when using essential oils.
- Do not use essential oils while on medication; the oils might interfere with the medicine.
- After an application of citrus oils on the skin, avoid sunbathing, saunas, and hot baths, to prevent skin damage.

HANDLING OF OILS

- Essential oils spilled on furniture will remove the finish; therefore, be careful when handling the bottles.
- Store essential oils in brown-colored glass bottles and keep them in a dark, cool place.
- Always use a glass dropper when measuring drops of essential oil.
- Keep all bottles tightly closed to prevent the oils from evaporating and oxidizing.
- Always store essential oils out of reach and out of sight of children.

HELPFUL MEASUREMENTS

100 drops=1 teaspoon=5 ml
300 drops=1 tablespoon=15 ml
600 drops=1 ounce=30 ml
4 ounces=120 ml
4 ounces (dry)=100 g

CHAPTER 4

THE POWER OF THE MIND

✿ ✿ ✿

THE INCREDIBLE HUMAN brain is the most complex structure of living cells known in the universe. It weighs approximately three pounds (1.35 kilo), consumes about 20% of the body's oxygen intake, and contains up to 100 billion neurons and a greater number of glial cells that nourish and service the neurons. Unlike the other brains in the animal kingdom, the human brain possesses the ability of a higher consciousness to think logically, reason, and plan; great creative imagination to envision what is not yet in existence; and the capability to take action to carry out a vision until it becomes reality.

The brain can provide a person with the ability to generate extraordinary thoughts and ideas to build magnificent structures, machinery, equipment, and tools; devise clever ways to overcome obstacles to make life easier; trigger the emotions of love, compassion, and warmth; provide care and comfort for the sick and needy. On the other hand, the brain can help develop and produce the most disastrous weapons of war, which, when they are used, bring great pain, suffering, and annihilation to large numbers of people and other living things. Each one

of us chooses the purposes we want to use our brain for. To be productive and constructive, or destructive—the choice is ours to make.

Firewalking, the astounding act of walking on hot, burning coals, dates back 2,500 years. It is a deeply ingrained tradition in certain cultures of China, Japan, Tibet, and India. Later, firewalking spread to Europe and other parts of the world.

How can a person walk on burning coals that reach temperatures as high as 1200–1300°F (500–600°C), without getting burned? When a yogi sits on a board laden with protruding sharp nails why doesn't he receive even a single scratch? And if a yogi in a meditative state is buried alive for several hours or days, how is it possible to find him alive when he is dug up?

Can the power of the mind produce these phenomenal acts that appear to defy the laws of science?

The answer is yes!

In 1964, noted writer and editor Norman Cousins became ill with ankylosing spondylitis, an excruciatingly debilitating disease that attacks the connective tissue and fuses the joints together. His spine was disintegrating and he could hardly move his jaw to open his mouth. Cousins was given a one in 500 chance to live, but the specialist who examined him cautioned Cousins that he hadn't heard of anyone who had previously survived the disease.

Alarmed by the prognosis, Cousins researched extensively the deleterious effects stress and negative emotions have on the body. He decided to take responsibility for his recovery and pursue a positive attitude. He discontinued his pain medication and began to practice "laughter therapy," watching comedy films and reading humorous books.

Cousins improved dramatically. After only four months he miraculously returned to work full-time.

On another occasion, Cousins made an experiment to determine the effect that inner feelings have on the cells of the immune system. He took a sample of blood, waited five minutes, then took another sample. Before taking the second sample, he put himself in a state of joyous excitement and elation. He visualized a peaceful world and people being kind and getting along with one another.

The results of the tests were amazing. He found an average increase of 50% of immune system cells in the second sample: B cells, T cells, cytotoxic cells, and N K cells.

In 1979, Cousins wrote an inspirational best-selling book, *Anatomy of an Illness,* crediting positive thinking for his recovery. Holding the belief that emotions play a major role in determining a person's state of health, Cousins' book conveys the impor-

tance of taking responsibility for the outcome of your life.

Jason Winters was living a life of adventure and excitement. He crossed the Canadian Rockies in a hot-air balloon, canoed 2,000 miles (3,200 km) down the Mackenzie River, crossed the Sahara Desert by camel, tested seat belts by crashing into brick walls, and performed as a stunt man in the movies. During this time, he smoked 30 cigarettes daily and drank rye whiskey heavily once a week.

One day Winters noticed a tumor on the side of his neck. He hoped it would go away, but it kept getting larger. The growth was attached to his jugular vein and wrapped around his carotid artery. Winters was diagnosed as having terminal cancer, but he refused surgery.

Driven by a great will to live and his love for life, Winters stopped his bad habits and completely changed his lifestyle. He started a program in an attempt to reverse his illness. With a positive mindset, great hope, determination, and by taking a mixture of herbs daily, he miraculously regained his health and was back at work in nine weeks. Winters' remarkable recovery is fully detailed in his book, *The Jason Winters Story.*

On May 6, 1954, Roger Bannister, a 25-year-old British track runner, shocked the sports world. He broke the four-minute-mile barrier in 3:59.4 minutes at a race in Oxford, England. Until the day Bannister broke the record, it had been a well-accepted fact that no human being could run a mile in less than four minutes. However, within a few months after this belief was shattered by Bannister, other track runners were also able to break the four-minute mile. Since then, it is estimated that over 400 runners have succeeded in duplicating or bettering Bannister's accomplishment.

In the 1976 World Olympic games the Russians dominated by winning more medals than any other country. At first they were suspected of using steroid drugs. It was later discovered that the Russians engaged in mind conditioning of their athletes.

Athletes who condition their minds for peak performance during sport events enter a state of intense concentration brought on by profound changes in the brain. The left brain hemisphere erupts with what is called *alpha waves*, indicative of a trance-like state. This results in the left brain becoming relaxed and the right brain taking control. In addition to athletes, many successful musicians, entertainers, and performers experience this state when they are engaged in their performances. It is known that 60–90% of an athlete's sports performance is due to the conditioning of the mind.

VISUALIZATION

Visualization is an innate process of using our thoughts and imagination to create a picture in our mind of a goal we are seeking to accomplish. We practice mental imagery regularly on many occasions without realizing it. Everything we do in life originates in the mind as a thought or a vision. We are visualizing when we imagine ourselves living in a new house or visiting a new country. Often our ideas progressively develop into a tangible goal. This process is the vital doorway that enables us to see and plan for what we want in life.

When we fail continuously without learning from our mistakes, it is due to our conditioned, deep-seated negative feelings imprinted from our past, which we unconsciously use to sabotage ourselves, creating difficulties, problems, limitations, and ultimately leading to more failures. Acknowledging this process can help overcome deep-rooted problems, which require an extraordinary amount of will and determination to be successfully resolved.

When wanting to achieve a specific goal, it is important first to make sure it is realistic and attainable. Then support your goal with an outline of a plan of action and the time frame in which you would like to see it come to fruition. Remember, the major factor that will determine your success hinges upon the strength of your desire to achieve—your determination.

INTUITION

Everyone has intuition, though it is more developed and used by some individuals than others. Intuition is a strong feeling of inner wisdom, an inner voice providing us with valuable information and insight. Its role is vital, yet the messages are frequently ignored by those who do not understand or trust it.

Dreams have been recognized as a source

of intuitional insight since early times. Examples abound of ideas dreams have provided to inventors, writers, artists, and other creative people.

Elias Howe tried unsuccessfully for years to invent a machine that would sew clothing. One night he dreamed he had been captured by members of a tribe who threw spears at him. Each spear had a hole near its sharp tip and would repeatedly bounce up and down off the ground. When Howe awoke, he realized the dream had provided him with the necessary input to perfect what became known as the sewing machine.

Niels Bohr dreamed of a day at the races and realized that the lanes at the racetrack were an example of the specific orbits electrons follow around atomic nuclei. Bohr later won the Nobel Prize for the discovery of the quantum theory.

Robert Louis Stevenson credited his dreams for many story ideas, including the key characters of Dr. Jekyll and Mr. Hyde. Samuel Taylor Coleridge said he dictated *The Rime of the Ancient Mariner* from a dream.

However beneficial intuition is, it is best not to rely on it solely for decision making, without giving the issue at hand further thought. Since intuition emanates from the right side of the brain, it should be balanced by processing the input additionally through the left side of the brain, where logic and reason predominate. In other words, don't run out and invest all your money in the stock market because of a hunch you felt was your intuition.

REFLECTION

Our thoughts, hopes and actions of today play a key role in contributing to the shape of our world of tomorrow. It is vital to probe ourselves periodically to assess and evaluate our general purpose and direction in life. Just as a captain who navigates a ship, we must know our position and steer our course towards our desired destination.

INTROSPECTION

Many of us are so absorbed in our work and daily affairs that we seldom take the time to examine our inner thoughts and feelings or evaluate the extent to which we honor our promises, commitments, and responsibilities to relatives, business associates, friends, acquaintances, and others in our life.

MOTIVES FOR OUR ACTIONS

Two people can perform the same act but yet each person can have a different motive for doing so. For example: One woman helps a sick relative because she anticipates receiving a large inheritance in reward for her actions. Another woman helps a sick relative out of compassion and caring for a human being, and seeks no reward in return. It is important to examine our motives of why we do things and what we expect in return.

Improvement

Every day we have the opportunity to acquire additional knowledge, think of new ideas, improve ourself, and make life more meaningful. Perhaps the greatest chance we have to improve, which few people take advantage of, is giving consideration when we are offered constructive criticism. Everyone seems to enjoy being complimented, but hardly anyone is receptive to criticism.

There are people who care about us and point out key observations to try and help us. It takes a special caring person who has the courage to do so, sometimes at the risk of offending someone and losing a friendship. Be grateful and appreciative, accept the criticism in a positive way. Reflect on how this valuable advice can help you improve. Even if you feel the criticism is only 10% valid, at least reflect on the 10%, don't ignore it.

This course of contemplation can prove to be an invaluable tool as you progress up the path of life.

Loving Oneself

Many people engage in self-destructive behavior: overeating, smoking, or excessive alcohol intake. This may be a result of negative childhood conditioning or could have been acquired over the years to deal with a lifestyle that is overly stressful and frustrating.

Free yourself by relinquishing habits that are harmful, replacing them with activities and behavior that give you great joy, satisfaction, and help you feel good about yourself.

Appreciation

In this fast-paced life we rush through time, on many occasions failing to acknowledge inwardly and outwardly the things and people we have to be thankful for. Take time out to feel appreciative for all you have. Give thanks for having food, shelter, clothing, friends and family, and even a pet. One cannot experience the joy of true happiness while taking the necessities of life for granted.

Meditation

Meditation relaxes the metabolism to a lower point than sleep, as the body gains a deep, concentrated level of rest. The rate of breathing and the amount of oxygen intake is decreased and so are the blood pressure and heartbeat rate.

Meditation is a quieting of the conscious mind. The stillness of this state allows deeper levels of relaxation and peacefulness to be attained. It enables a greater ability to focus and allow thoughts to develop. This is a state in which the mind does not engage in judgment or analysis. There is awareness of all thoughts that arise, but these thoughts are allowed to pass by without being analyzed. People who practice meditation regularly respond to stressful situations more effectively and thus decrease stress levels and anxiety dramatically.

The benefits of meditation are cumulative

and offer profound improvement to physical and emotional health. It is important to practice these exercises regularly to achieve best results.

RELAXATION

In recent years, deep relaxation, visualization, and meditation exercises have become more popularly practiced in the Western world, and people have benefited immensely from these various techniques. By incorporating the essential oil formulas, the results obtained are even more profound, especially for people who have difficulty entering a relaxed state.

GUIDELINES TO PREPARE FOR RELAXATION

• Find a peaceful and comfortable place to relax.
• Make sure you will not be disturbed by the telephone, doorbell, people entering the room, or noisy pets.
• The room temperature should be warm.
• Soft music in the background can enhance relaxation.

• Determine the easiest and most natural method to relax:
    1) Listening to a relaxation tape
    2) Guiding yourself with images
    3) Using thoughts to create a state of mind
• Relaxation position: Sitting comfortably in a well-supported chair with your back straight and feet flat on the floor, or lying in a supine position.

RELAXATION EXERCISE

Take a deep breath. As you exhale, close your eyes. Continue breathing slowly and fully. (Pause.) Scan your body and pinpoint tense areas. Focus on sending deep relaxation to each individual area. (Pause.) With each inhalation, you relax further. As you exhale, the tension releases and exits your body, enabling you to feel peaceful and serene. Let go of any extraneous thoughts and give yourself permission to experience inner peace and stillness. (Pause.) Focus on your breathing. Begin to count down slowly from 20 to 1, taking a full breath with each number. Allow yourself to enter a deeper level of tranquility. Detach yourself from the outside world until you cease to be aware of it.

FORMULAS

Before using any of the formulas, please be sure to have read carefully chapters 2 and 3.

APPRECIATION

It is important to appreciate everything we have in life. It is unfortunate that too many people wait for their deathbeds or for a tragedy to occur before experiencing feelings of contrition and regret at not having enjoyed the closeness of loved ones.

• Choose one of these methods: application, diffusor, mist spray; select and use a formula.
• Do the relaxation exercise on page 24. Allow yourself to reach a peaceful and quiet state. Think of the special people you know. Fill out the Appreciation Worksheet. Repeat this exercise whenever possible. Each session should be 20–30 minutes.

APPLICATION

Apply one of these formulas to the upper chest and back of the neck until the oil is fully absorbed into the skin. Breathe in the vapors deeply.

Ylang-Ylang	4 drops		Sandalwood	4 drops
Allspice	3 drops		Bergamot	3 drops
Vanilla	3 drops		Geranium	3 drops
Carrier Oil	2 teaspoons		Carrier Oil	2 teaspoons
• • • • • •			• • • • • •	
Litsea Cubeba	3 drops		Bois de Rose	3 drops
Palmarosa	3 drops		Anise	3 drops
Neroli	2 drops		Ylang-Ylang	3 drops
Labdanum	2 drops		Cedarwood (Atlas)	1 drop
Carrier Oil	2 teaspoons		Carrier Oil	2 teaspoons
• • • • • •			• • • • • •	
Frankincense	3 drops		Patchouli	3 drops
Vanilla	3 drops		Bois de Rose	3 drops
Orange	3 drops		Lime	2 drops
Sandalwood	1 drop		Clove	2 drops
Carrier Oil	2 teaspoons		Carrier Oil	2 teaspoons

Vanilla	3 drops		Labdanum	5 drops
Bergamot	3 drops		Allspice	3 drops
Neroli	2 drops		Peppermint	2 drops
Cumin	2 drops		Carrier Oil	2 teaspoons
Carrier Oil	2 teaspoons			

DIFFUSOR

Depending on the type of diffusor you have, place the essential oils on the diffusor pad or in the glass bottle to disperse the aroma into the air.

Ylang-Ylang	30%		Ylang-Ylang	25%
Bois de Rose	30%		Palmarosa	25%
Orange	20%		Citronella	25%
Clove	20%		Frankincense	25%

• • • • • •   • • • • • •

Lavender	50%		Allspice	30%
Petitgrain	20%		Citronella	30%
Allspice	20%		Geranium	30%
Bergamot	10%		Bergamot	10%

MIST SPRAYS

Fill a fine-mist spray bottle with purified water, then add the essential oils. Tighten the cap and shake well. Mist numerous times and breathe in the vapors deeply.

Bergamot	50 drops		Lime	40 drops
Geranium	40 drops		Lavender	30 drops
Bois de Rose	40 drops		Geranium	30 drops
Sandalwood	20 drops		Ylang-Ylang	25 drops
Pure Water	4 ounces		Cedarwood (Atlas)	25 drops
			Pure Water	4 ounces

• • • • • •   • • • • • •

Frankincense	40 drops		Lavender	50 drops
Petitgrain	40 drops		Ylang-Ylang	50 drops
Mandarin	40 drops		Citronella	30 drops
Anise	30 drops		Sandalwood	20 drops
Pure Water	4 ounces		Pure Water	4 ounces

Allspice	40 drops		Bergamot	40 drops
Lavender	40 drops		Citronella	40 drops
Frankincense	40 drops		Bay	40 drops
Lemon	20 drops		Sandalwood	30 drops
Palmarosa	10 drops		Pure Water	4 ounces
Pure Water	4 ounces			

APPRECIATION WORKSHEET*

I wish to spend more time with:

1._____

2._____

3._____

4._____

5._____

6._____

7._____

I have made it my priority to set aside time from my busy schedule in order to be with the people I care about. Here are the specific day(s), week(s), or month(s) I will dedicate to each person:

1._____

2._____

3._____

4._____

5._____

6._____

7._____

Please make a copy of this worksheet and fill it out.

DREAMS

These formulas will help you recall your dreams. If you have difficulty obtaining results on the first application, repeat it for several nights.
- Apply one of the formulas before going to sleep.
- Place a pen or pencil, and paper, next to your bed to record the details.

APPLICATION

Apply one of these formulas to the upper chest and back of the neck until the oil is fully absorbed into the skin. Breathe in the vapors deeply.

Helichrysum	4 drops		Cedarwood (Atlas)	3 drops
Basil (Sweet)	3 drops		Cinnamon Leaf	3 drops
Tangerine	3 drops		Nutmeg	2 drops
Carrier Oil	2 teaspoons		Rosemary	2 drops
			Carrier Oil	2 teaspoons

• • • • • •

Frankincense	3 drops		Sandalwood	2 drops
Lemon	3 drops		Geranium	2 drops
Basil (Sweet)	3 drops		Lemon	2 drops
Sea Buckthorn	3 drops		Neroli	2 drops
Carrier Oil	2 teaspoons		Rosemary	2 drops
			Carrier Oil	2 teaspoons

IMPROVEMENT

- Choose one of these methods: application, diffusor, or mist spray; select and use a formula.
- Do the relaxation exercise on page 24. Allow yourself to reach an inner peaceful and quiet state, then reflect on specific changes you have to make in your life so you can improve yourself. Fill out the Improvement Worksheet to better organize your thoughts. Repeat this exercise as many times as you feel necessary. Each session should be 20–30 minutes.

APPLICATION

Apply one of these formulas to the upper chest and back of the neck until the oil is fully absorbed into the skin. Breathe in the vapors deeply.

Litsea Cubeba	4 drops		Spruce	4 drops
Cardamom	3 drops		Vanilla	3 drops
Cedarwood (Atlas)	3 drops		Grapefruit	3 drops
Carrier Oil	2 teaspoons		Carrier Oil	2 teaspoons

• • • • • •

Sandalwood	5 drops		Elemi	3 drops
Lemongrass	3 drops		Basil (Sweet)	3 drops
Pepper (Black)	2 drops		Geranium	2 drops
Carrier Oil	2 teaspoons		Palmarosa	2 drops
			Carrier Oil	2 teaspoons

• • • • • •

Bois de Rose	4 drops		Litsea Cubeba	4 drops
Cedarwood (Atlas)	3 drops		Vanilla	3 drops
Cardamom	3 drops		Sandalwood	3 drops
Carrier Oil	2 teaspoons		Carrier Oil	2 teaspoons

DIFFUSOR

Depending on the type of diffusor you have, place the essential oils on the diffusor pad or in the glass bottle to disperse the aroma into the air.

Grapefruit	40%		Bois de Rose	40%
Lime	30%		Litsea Cubeba	30%
Frankincense	30%		Geranium	20%
			Ginger	10%

• • • • • •

Litsea Cubeba	50%		Geranium	30%
Spruce	30%		Frankincense	30%
Basil (Sweet)	20%		Orange	30%
			Pepper (Black)	10%

MIST SPRAYS

Fill a fine-mist spray bottle with purified water, then add the essential oils. Tighten the cap and shake well. Mist numerous times and breathe in the vapors deeply.

Bois de Rose	50 drops		Lime	50 drops
Cardamom	40 drops		Geranium	30 drops
Lemongrass	40 drops		Orange	30 drops
Sandalwood	20 drops		Basil (Sweet)	20 drops
Pure Water	4 ounces		Ginger	20 drops
			Pure Water	4 ounces

• • • • • •

• • • • • •

Tangerine	50 drops		Frankincense	50 drops
Cedarwood (Atlas)	50 drops		Spruce	50 drops
Spruce	50 drops		Palmarosa	50 drops
Pure Water	4 ounces		Pure Water	4 ounces

IMPROVEMENT WORKSHEET*

Changes I have to make: _____

_____

_____

_____

_____

_____

Plan of action for each change: _____

_____

_____

_____

_____

_____

Please make a copy of this worksheet and fill it out.

INTROSPECTION

- Choose one of these methods: application, diffusor, or mist spray; select and use a formula.
- Do the relaxation exercise on page 24. Allow yourself to reach a peaceful, quiet state. Then take a closer look at yourself. On a personal level, compare how your daily actions measure up to your moral values and the principles you stand for. On an interpersonal level, examine how you honor your promises, commitments, and responsibilities to the people in your life. To help organize your thoughts, fill out the Introspection Worksheet. Repeat this exercise as many times as you feel necessary. Each session should be 20–30 minutes.

APPLICATION

Apply one of these formulas to the upper chest and the back of the neck, until the oil has been fully absorbed into the skin. Breathe in the vapors deeply.

Elemi	3 drops	Basil (Sweet)	3 drops
Frankincense	3 drops	Sandalwood	3 drops
Lemon	2 drops	Pepper (Black)	2 drops
Tangerine	2 drops	Orange	2 drops
Carrier Oil	2 teaspoons	Carrier Oil	2 teaspoons
• • • • • •		• • • • • •	
Pepper (Black)	3 drops	Myrrh	3 drops
Spruce	3 drops	Cypress	3 drops
Frankincense	2 drops	Labdanum	3 drops
Lemon	2 drops	Tangerine	1 drop
Carrier Oil	2 teaspoons	Carrier Oil	2 teaspoons
• • • • • •		• • • • • •	
Petitgrain	3 drops	Cedarwood (Atlas)	3 drops
Sandalwood	3 drops	Basil (Sweet)	3 drops
Cajeput	2 drops	Spikenard	2 drops
Myrrh	2 drops	Rosemary	2 drops
Carrier Oil	2 teaspoons	Carrier Oil	2 teaspoons
• • • • • •		• • • • • •	
Vetiver	4 drops	Sandalwood	4 drops
Cypress	3 drops	Bois de Rose	3 drops
Lemongrass	3 drops	Nutmeg	2 drops
Carrier Oil	2 teaspoons	Clove	1 drop
		Carrier Oil	2 teaspoons

Peru Balsam	3 drops	Spruce	3 drops
Bois de Rose	3 drops	Bois de Rose	3 drops
Myrrh	2 drops	Petitgrain	2 drops
Rosemary	2 drops	Cedarwood (Atlas)	2 drops
Carrier Oil	2 teaspoons	Carrier Oil	2 teaspoons

DIFFUSOR

Depending on the type of diffusor you have, place the essential oils on the diffusor pad or in the glass bottle to disperse the aroma into the air.

Frankincense	50%	Bois de Rose	40%
Spruce	50%	Petitgrain	40%
		Juniper Berry	20%

• • • • • •

Lime	40%	Petitgrain	50%
Tangerine	30%	Basil (Sweet)	20%
Cypress	30%	Allspice	20%
		Rosemary	10%

MIST SPRAYS

Fill a fine-mist spray bottle with purified water, then add the essential oils. Tighten the cap and shake well. Mist numerous times and breathe in the vapors deeply.

Frankincense	50 drops	Cedarwood (Atlas)	45 drops
Vetiver	50 drops	Lime	45 drops
Orange	50 drops	Elemi	40 drops
Pure Water	4 ounces	Grapefruit	20 drops
		Pure Water	4 ounces

• • • • • •

Bay	50 drops	Frankincense	40 drops
Sandalwood	50 drops	Nutmeg	40 drops
Cajeput	30 drops	Copaiba	30 drops
Mandarin	20 drops	Lime	30 drops
Pure Water	4 ounces	Orange	10 drops
		Pure Water	4 ounces

INTROSPECTION WORKSHEET #1*

Insights on a personal level: _____

_____

_____

_____

Planned changes: _____

_____

_____

_____

Actions to be taken: _____

_____

_____

INTROSPECTION WORKSHEET #2*

Insights on an interpersonal level: _____

_____

_____

_____

Planned changes: _____

_____

_____

_____

Actions to be taken: _____

_____

_____

*Please make a copy of these worksheets and fill them out.

INTUITION

If you have a decision to make and need guidance by looking within, these intuition formulas will help relax your mind to assist you in the appropriate course of action.

- Choose one of these methods: application, diffusor, or mist spray; select and use a formula.
- Do the relaxation exercise on page 24. Allow yourself to reach a peaceful and quiet state. Clear your mind of all extraneous thoughts, and focus on the guidance you are seeking. Repeat this exercise once daily if possible, for 20–30 minutes. It may take several days to get the insight you are looking for. Use the Intuition Worksheet to better organize your thoughts, and record your insight.
- After you have received the answers, ponder the input with one of the mental concentration formulas.

APPLICATION

Apply one of these formulas to the upper chest and the back of the neck, until the oil is fully absorbed into the skin. Breathe in the vapors deeply.

Frankincense	4 drops	Ginger	3 drops
Elemi	3 drops	Spruce	3 drops
Lime	3 drops	Lemon	2 drops
Carrier Oil	2 teaspoons	Peru Balsam	2 drops
		Carrier Oil	2 teaspoons

• • • • • •

• • • • • •

Bay	4 drops	Citronella	3 drops
Copaiba	3 drops	Litsea Cubeba	3 drops
Neroli	3 drops	Frankincense	3 drops
Carrier Oil	2 teaspoons	Sandalwood	1 drop
		Carrier Oil	2 teaspoons

• • • • • •

• • • • • •

Elemi	4 drops	Guaiacwood	3 drops
Cedarwood (Atlas)	4 drops	Labdanum	3 drops
Neroli	2 drops	Rosemary	2 drops
Carrier Oil	2 teaspoons	Citronella	2 drops
		Carrier Oil	2 teaspoons

Chamomile (Roman)	5 drops		Fir Needles	3 drops
Orange	5 drops		Chamomile (Roman)	3 drops
Carrier Oil	2 teaspoons		Spruce	2 drops
			Basil (Sweet)	2 drops
			Carrier Oil	2 teaspoons

DIFFUSOR

Depending on the type of diffusor you have, place the essential oils on the diffusor pad or in the glass bottle to disperse the aroma into the air.

Frankincense	50%		Grapefruit	50%
Spruce	30%		Ginger	20%
Lemon	20%		Tangerine	20%
			Rosemary	10%

• • • • • •

Tangerine	40%		Bay	25%
Frankincense	40%		Lime	25%
Ginger	20%		Basil (Sweet)	25%
			Petitgrain	25%

• • • • • •

Tangerine	40%		Lemon	50%
Fir Needles	40%		Chamomile (Roman)	50%
Basil (Sweet)	20%			

MIST SPRAYS

Fill a fine-mist spray bottle with purified water, then add the essential oils. Tighten the cap and shake well. Mist numerous times and breathe in the vapors deeply.

Frankincense	50 drops		Lemongrass	40 drops
Myrtle	50 drops		Bergamot	30 drops
Lemon	25 drops		Copaiba	30 drops
Bay	25 drops		Ginger	25 drops
Pure Water	4 ounces		Vetiver	25 drops
			Pure Water	4 ounces

Myrtle	30 drops		Litsea Cubeba	50 drops
Tangerine	30 drops		Frankincense	40 drops
Chamomile (Roman)	30 drops		Nutmeg	20 drops
Allspice	30 drops		Ginger	30 drops
Cedarwood (Atlas)	30 drops		Mandarin	10 drops
Pure Water	4 ounces		Pure Water	4 ounces

INTUITION WORKSHEET*

I am seeking inner guidance for the following decsion: _____

_____

_____

_____

Specific insights: _____

_____

_____

OPTIONS

List options, then explore each one individually to determine which is the

best.

1._____

2._____

3._____

4._____

Plan of action:

_____

_____

_____

_____

*Please make a copy of this worksheet and fill it out.

LOVING YOURSELF

- Choose one of these methods: application, aroma lamp, diffusor, or mist spray; select and use a formula.
- Do the relaxation exercise on page 24. Allow yourself to reach a peaceful and quiet state. Reflect on the things you enjoy doing that bring great satisfaction, make you feel good, and at the same time are beneficial for your well-being. Repeat this exercise as often as possible. Each session should be 20–30 minutes.

APPLICATION

Apply one of these formulas to the upper chest and the back of the neck, until the oil is fully absorbed into the skin. Breathe in the vapors deeply.

Spruce	4 drops		Ylang-Ylang	4 drops
Sandalwood	3 drops		Orange	3 drops
Vanilla	3 drops		Sandalwood	3 drops
Carrier Oil	2 teaspoons		Carrier Oil	2 teaspoons
• • • • • •			• • • • • •	
Sandalwood	4 drops		Bergamot	5 drops
Vanilla	3 drops		Copaiba	3 drops
Grapefruit	3 drops		Neroli	2 drops
Carrier Oil	2 teaspoons		Carrier Oil	2 teaspoons
• • • • • •			• • • • • •	
Cedarwood (Atlas)	3 drops		Spruce	4 drops
Clove	3 drops		Frankincense	3 drops
Tangerine	3 drops		Ylang-Ylang	3 drops
Myrrh	1 drop		Carrier Oil	2 teaspoons
Carrier Oil	2 teaspoons		• • • • • •	
• • • • • •				
Copaiba	5 drops		Vanilla	4 drops
Tangerine	3 drops		Ylang-Ylang	4 drops
Juniper Berry	2 drops		Juniper Berry	2 drops
Carrier Oil	2 teaspoons		Carrier Oil	2 teaspoons

Labdanum	5 drops	Vanilla	4 drops
Allspice	3 drops	Labdanum	4 drops
Lavender	2 drops	Rose	2 drops
Carrier Oil	2 teaspoons	Carrier Oil	2 teaspoons

AROMA LAMP

Place water in the container, add the essential oils, then heat. Inhale the vapors deeply.

Sandalwood	8 drops	Ylang-Ylang	7 drops
Spruce	8 drops	Frankincense	7 drops
Bergamot	4 drops	Juniper Berry	6 drops

• • • • • •   • • • • • •

Copaiba	8 drops	Ylang-Ylang	7 drops
Bergamot	8 drops	Cumin	5 drops
Myrrh	4 drops	Orange	5 drops
		Cedarwood (Atlas)	3 drops

• • • • • •   • • • • • •

Spruce	8 drops	Sandalwood	8 drops
Petitgrain	6 drops	Ginger	4 drops
Juniper Berry	6 drops	Grapefruit	4 drops
		Clove	4 drops

DIFFUSOR

Depending on the type of diffusor you have, place the essential oils on the diffusor pad or in the glass bottle to disperse the aroma into the air.

Ylang-Ylang	40%	Frankincense	40%
Juniper Berry	30%	Bergamot	40%
Clove	30%	Orange	20%

• • • • • •   • • • • • •

Bergamot	40%	Petitgrain	40%
Spruce	40%	Juniper Berry	30%
Ylang-Ylang	20%	Spruce	30%

Grapefruit	50%		Lime	50%
Clove	30%		Mandarin	30%
Citronella	20%		Ylang-Ylang	20%

• • • • • •   • • • • • •

Ylang-Ylang	50%		Grapefruit	30%
Tangerine	50%		Petitgrain	30%
			Ginger	20%
			Ylang-Ylang	20%

MIST SPRAYS

Fill a fine-mist spray bottle with purified water, then add the essential oils. Tighten the cap and shake well. Mist numerous times and breathe in the vapors deeply.

Ylang-Ylang	50 drops		Grapefruit	60 drops
Sandalwood	50 drops		Peru Balsam	60 drops
Clove	30 drops		Juniper Berry	30 drops
Citronella	20 drops		Pure Water	4 ounces
Pure Water	4 ounces			

• • • • • •   • • • • • •

Frankincense	50 drops		Allspice	40 drops
Cedarwood (Atlas)	50 drops		Ylang-Ylang	30 drops
Tangerine	50 drops		Spruce	30 drops
Pure Water	4 ounces		Myrrh	30 drops
			Orange	20 drops
			Pure Water	4 ounces

• • • • • •   • • • • • •

Bergamot	50 drops		Cedarwood (Atlas)	50 drops
Copaiba	50 drops		Myrrh	40 drops
Peru Balsam	50 drops		Mandarin	40 drops
Pure Water	4 ounces		Clove	20 drops
			Pure Water	4 ounces

Peru Balsam	50 drops		Lemon	60 drops
Citronella	50 drops		Peru Balsam	60 drops
Tangerine	50 drops		Bois de Rose	30 drops
Pure Water	4 ounces		Pure Water	4 ounces

MEDITATION

The meditative state not only relaxes the body, but it rejuvenates the mind and nervous system also.

- Choose one of these methods: application, diffusor, or mist spray; select and use a formula.
- Do the relaxation exercise on page 24. Allow yourself to reach a peaceful and quiet state of mind and maintain this level of calmness for 20–30 minutes. Practice as often as you can.

APPLICATION

Apply one of these formulas to the upper chest and the back of the neck, until the oil is fully absorbed into the skin. Breathe the vapors deeply.

Frankincense	5 drops		Elemi	5 drops
Orange	5 drops		Litsea Cubeba	5 drops
Carrier Oil	2 teaspoons		Carrier Oil	2 teaspoons
• • • • • •			• • • • • •	
Copaiba	5 drops		Cedarwood (Atlas)	5 drops
Lemon	3 drops		Spruce	5 drops
Nutmeg	2 drops		Carrier Oil	2 teaspoons
Carrier Oil	2 teaspoons		• • • • • •	
• • • • • •				
Sandalwood	4 drops		Peru Balsam	4 drops
Basil (Sweet)	4 drops		Nutmeg	3 drops
Lavender	2 drops		Spikenard	3 drops
Carrier Oil	2 teaspoons		Carrier Oil	2 teaspoons
• • • • • •			• • • • • •	
Labdanum	6 drops		Guaiacwood	5 drops
Clary Sage	4 drops		Tangerine	5 drops
Carrier Oil	2 teaspoons		Carrier Oil	2 teaspoons

Guaiacwood	5 drops	Peru Balsam	5 drops
Petitgrain	3 drops	Orange	3 drops
Frankincense	2 drops	Cumin	2 drops
Carrier Oil	2 teaspoons	Carrier Oil	2 teaspoons

DIFFUSOR

Depending on the type of diffusor you have, place the essential oils on the diffusor pad or in the glass bottle to disperse the aroma into the air.

Frankincense	50%	Lavender	50%
Orange	30%	Basil (Sweet)	25%
Petitgrain	20%	Anise	25%

• • • • • •

Litsea Cubeba	50%	Tangerine	50%
Nutmeg	25%	Frankincense	30%
Clary Sage	25%	Basil (Sweet)	20%

• • • • • •

Mandarin	50%	Orange	50%
Lavender	50%	Spruce	30%
		Nutmeg	20%

MIST SPRAYS

Fill a fine-mist spray bottle with purified water, then add the essential oils. Tighten the cap and shake well. Mist numerous times and breathe in the vapors deeply.

Frankincense	75 drops	Sandalwood	50 drops
Orange	50 drops	Frankincense	50 drops
Nutmeg	25 drops	Spruce	50 drops
Pure Water	4 ounces	Pure Water	4 ounces

• • • • • •

Cedarwood (Atlas)	60 drops	Lavender	60 drops
Litsea Cubeba	60 drops	Vetiver	50 drops
Clary Sage	30 drops	Anise	40 drops
Pure Water	4 ounces	Pure Water	4 ounces

Elemi	60 drops	Copaiba	70 drops
Litsea Cubeba	50 drops	Orange	50 drops
Petitgrain	40 drops	Frankincense	30 drops
Pure Water	4 ounces	Pure Water	4 ounces

MENTAL CONCENTRATION

With the advent of high-tech devices, such as the computer and calculator, people seem to depend more on machines to do their figuring than on their own minds.

These formulas help promote the concentration needed for developing new thoughts and ideas, for planning, creativity, and problem solving. The mental concentration blends can be a valuable tool when used in conjunction with the input derived from the intuition exercises.

• Choose one of these methods: application, aroma lamp, baths, diffusor, mist spray; select and use a formula. Afterwards, spend 20 minutes in a quiet, comfortable place.

APPLICATION

Apply one of these formulas to the back of the neck, chest, and temple area until the oil is fully absorbed into the skin. Breathe in the vapors deeply.

Spearmint	4 drops	Grapefruit	4 drops
Tangerine	4 drops	Copaiba	3 drops
Cedarwood (Atlas)	2 drops	Hyssop Decumbens	3 drops
Sesame	2 teaspoons	Sesame	2 teaspoons

• • • • • •

Spearmint	4 drops	Bergamot	4 drops
Ginger	4 drops	Orange	2 drops
Sandalwood	2 drops	Coriander	2 drops
Sesame	2 teaspoons	Copaiba	2 drops
		Sesame	2 teaspoons

• • • • • •

Rosemary	4 drops	Grapefruit	4 drops
Bergamot	4 drops	Bay	4 drops
Clove	2 drops	Copaiba	2 drops
Sesame	2 teaspoons	Sesame	2 teaspoons

Juniper Berry	3 drops	Coriander	4 drops
Bergamot	3 drops	Lime	3 drops
Lime	3 drops	Sandalwood	3 drops
Rosemary	1 drop	Sesame	2 teaspoons
Sesame	2 teaspoons		

• • • • • • •

Peppermint	5 drops	Hyssop Decumbens	4 drops
Cedarwood (Atlas)	3 drops	Peppermint	4 drops
Eucalyptus	2 drops	Sandalwood	2 drops
Sesame	2 teaspoons	Sesame	2 teaspoons

AROMA LAMP

Place water in the container, add the essential oils, then heat. Inhale the vapors deeply.

Bay	10 drops	Lime	10 drops
Cedarwood (Atlas)	5 drops	Rosemary	10 drops
Orange	5 drops		

• • • • • • •

Spearmint	10 drops	Lemon	10 drops
Bergamot	7 drops	Patchouli	5 drops
Copaiba	3 drops	Clove	5 drops

• • • • • • •

Tangerine	10 drops	Grapefruit	15 drops
Cardamom	5 drops	Sandalwood	5 drops
Copaiba	5 drops		

• • • • • • •

Bergamot	10 drops	Clove	10 drops
Juniper Berry	5 drops	Ginger	5 drops
Eucalyptus	5 drops	Hyssop Decumbens	5 drops

• • • • • • •

Coriander	10 drops	Spearmint	10 drops
Cedarwood (Atlas)	5 drops	Citronella	5 drops
Lemon	5 drops	Copaiba	5 drops

BATHS

Fill the bathtub with water, as warm as you like. Mix the formula together, pour into the bathwater and disperse evenly throughout the tub. Breathe in the vapors deeply. Enjoy your bath for 30 minutes.

Spearmint	5 drops		Lavender	5 drops
Eucalyptus	4 drops		Lemon	5 drops
Orange	4 drops		Rosemary	5 drops
Hyssop Decumbens	2 drops		Carrier Oil	1 teaspoon
Carrier Oil	1 teaspoon			

• • • • • • (left) • • • • • • (right)

Spearmint	5 drops		Grapefruit	6 drops
Sandalwood	4 drops		Cedarwood (Atlas)	5 drops
Coriander	3 drops		Litsea Cubeba	4 drops
Hyssop Decumbens	3 drops		Carrier Oil	1 teaspoon
Carrier Oil	1 teaspoon			

• • • • • • (left) • • • • • • (right)

Peppermint	5 drops		Rosemary	5 drops
Copaiba	4 drops		Lemon	5 drops
Juniper Berry	3 drops		Bay	3 drops
Citronella	3 drops		Sandalwood	2 drops
Carrier Oil	1 teaspoon		Carrier Oil	1 teaspoon

• • • • • • (left) • • • • • • (right)

Tangerine	4 drops		Cardamom	5 drops
Cedarwood (Atlas)	4 drops		Litsea Cubeba	5 drops
Lemon	4 drops		Eucalyptus	3 drops
Rosemary	3 drops		Copaiba	2 drops
Carrier Oil	1 teaspoon		Carrier Oil	1 teaspoon

• • • • • • (left) • • • • • • (right)

Rosemary	5 drops		Lemon	5 drops
Pine	4 drops		Patchouli	4 drops
Fir Needles	3 drops		Juniper Berry	3 drops
Sandalwood	3 drops		Peppermint	3 drops
Carrier Oil	1 teaspoon		Carrier Oil	1 teaspoon

DIFFUSOR

Depending on the type of diffusor you have, place the essential oils on the diffusor pad or in the glass bottle to disperse the aroma into the air.

Peppermint	70%		Bergamot	50%
Cinnamon Leaf	30%		Spearmint	50%
• • • • • •			• • • • • •	
Peppermint	50%		Bay	35%
Copaiba	25%		Rosemary	35%
Bay	25%		Citronella	30%
• • • • • •			• • • • • •	
Hyssop Decumbens	50%		Cardamom	50%
Citronella	25%		Peppermint	30%
Lemon	25%		Cinnamon Leaf	20%
• • • • • •			• • • • • •	
Fir Needles	40%		Peppermint	70%
Lemon	20%		Tea Tree	30%
Petitgrain	20%			
Juniper Berry	20%			
• • • • • •			• • • • • •	
Spearmint	50%		Grapefruit	50%
Eucalyptus	25%		Clove	30%
Basil (Sweet)	25%		Litsea Cubeba	20%

MIST SPRAYS

Fill a fine-mist spray bottle with purified water and add the essential oils. Tighten the cap and shake well. Breathe in the vapors deeply.

Litsea Cubeba	40 drops		Grapefruit	50 drops
Sandalwood	40 drops		Copaiba	50 drops
Rosemary	40 drops		Orange	30 drops
Lemongrass	30 drops		Ginger	20 drops
Pure Water	4 ounces		Pure Water	4 ounces

Fir Needles	40 drops
Bay	40 drops
Coriander	40 drops
Sandalwood	30 drops
Pure Water	4 ounces

• • • • • • •

Peppermint	80 drops
Lemon	30 drops
Tea Tree	20 drops
Cedarwood (Atlas)	20 drops
Pure Water	4 ounces

• • • • • • •

Lemongrass	60 drops
Juniper Berry	30 drops
Copaiba	30 drops
Ginger	30 drops
Pure Water	4 ounces

• • • • • •

Bergamot	40 drops
Cardamom	30 drops
Lime	30 drops
Cypress	20 drops
Sage	15 drops
Sandalwood	15 drops
Pure Water	4 ounces

Bergamot	40 drops
Grapefruit	40 drops
Rosemary	40 drops
Copaiba	30 drops
Pure Water	4 ounces

• • • • • • •

Spearmint	70 drops
Cinnamon Leaf	40 drops
Coriander	20 drops
Copaiba	20 drops
Pure Water	4 ounces

• • • • • • •

Grapefruit	50 drops
Thyme	40 drops
Rosemary	20 drops
Sage	15 drops
Basil (Sweet)	15 drops
Sandalwood	10 drops
Pure Water	4 ounces

• • • • • • •

Lemon	50 drops
Rosemary	50 drops
Cedarwood (Atlas)	20 drops
Litsea Cubeba	15 drops
Basil (Sweet)	15 drops
Pure Water	4 ounces

MOTIVES FOR OUR ACTIONS

This exercise can be a valuable means of understanding how honest we are with ourselves to help us lessen inner conflicts and eventually create a state of inner peacefulness and well-being.

• Choose one of these methods: application, diffusor, or mist sprays; select and use a formula.

• Do the relaxation exercise on page 24. Allow yourself to reach a quiet state of mind. Then examine the actions you take and the motives behind them. Each session should be 20–30 minutes.

APPLICATION

Apply one of these formulas to the upper chest, back of the neck, and shoulders until the oil is fully absorbed into the skin. Breathe in the vapors deeply.

Spruce	4 drops	Bay	4 drops
Labdanum	4 drops	Tangerine	4 drops
Litsea Cubeba	2 drops	Patchouli	2 drops
Carrier Oil	2 teaspoons	Carrier Oil	2 teaspoons

• • • • • •

Geranium	4 drops	Copaiba	5 drops
Bois de Rose	3 drops	Pepper (Black)	3 drops
Sandalwood	3 drops	Tangerine	2 drops
Carrier Oil	2 teaspoons	Carrier Oil	2 teaspoons

• • • • • •

Peru Balsam	5 drops	Frankincense	4 drops
Lemon	5 drops	Cedarwood (Atlas)	4 drops
Carrier Oil	2 teaspoons	Spikenard	2 drops
		Carrier Oil	2 teaspoons

DIFFUSORS

Depending on the type of diffusor you have, place the essential oils on the diffusor pad or in the glass bottle to disperse the aroma into the air.

Spruce	50%	Tangerine	50%
Palmarosa	30%	Spruce	30%
Petitgrain	20%	Citronella	20%

• • • • • •

Bois de Rose	50%	Tangerine	40%
Lemon	30%	Bay	30%
Geranium	20%	Myrtle	30%

MIST SPRAYS

Fill a fine-mist spray bottle with purified water, then add the essential oils. Tighten the cap and shake well. Mist numerous times and breathe in the vapors deeply.

Spruce	50 drops		Peru Balsam	60 drops
Lemongrass	40 drops		Lemon	30 drops
Palmarosa	40 drops		Myrtle	30 drops
Cedarwood (Atlas)	20 drops		Spikenard	30 drops
Pure Water	4 ounces		Pure Water	4 ounces

• • • • • •   • • • • • •

Bois de Rose	60 drops		Tangerine	60 drops
Citronella	30 drops		Copaiba	40 drops
Tangerine	20 drops		Sandalwood	20 drops
Patchouli	20 drops		Bois de Rose	20 drops
Clove	20 drops		Vetiver	10 drops
Pure Water	4 ounces		Pure Water	4 ounces

REFLECTION

The path you have followed in prior years brought you to where you are now. The path you are on now will determine where you will be in life in future years.

Are you presently on the right path?

• Choose one of these methods: application, diffusor, or mist spray; select and use a formula.
• Do the relaxation exercise on page 24. Allow yourself to reach a peaceful and quiet state. Then, reflect on your path. Fill out the Reflection Worksheet to help organize your thoughts. Repeat this exercise as many times as you feel necessary. Each session should be 20–30 minutes.

APPLICATION

Apply one of these formulas to the back of the neck, upper chest, and temple area until the oil is fully absorbed into the skin. Breathe in the vapors deeply.

Litsea Cubeba	4 drops		Bay	4 drops
Pepper (Black)	3 drops		Lemongrass	4 drops
Cedarwood (Atlas)	3 drops		Patchouli	2 drops
Carrier Oil	2 teaspoons		Carrier Oil	2 teaspoons

Frankincense	4 drops		Elemi	4 drops
Spikenard	4 drops		Petitgrain	3 drops
Myrrh	2 drops		Hyssop Decumbens	3 drops
Carrier Oil	2 teaspoons		Carrier Oil	2 teaspoons

· · · · · ·

Spikenard	4 drops		Vetiver	4 drops
Orange	4 drops		Hyssop Decumbens	4 drops
Patchouli	2 drops		Chamomile (Roman)	2 drops
Carrier Oil	2 teaspoons		Carrier Oil	2 teaspoons

· · · · · ·

Fir Needles	4 drops		Lemon	4 drops
Litsea Cubeba	4 drops		Basil (Sweet)	4 drops
Frankincense	2 drops		Patchouli	2 drops
Carrier Oil	2 teaspoons		Carrier Oil	2 teaspoons

· · · · · ·

DIFFUSOR

Depending on the type of diffusor you have, place the essential oils on the diffusor pad or in the glass bottle to disperse the aroma into the air.

Frankincense	50%		Lemon	40%
Cinnamon Leaf	30%		Bay	40%
Fir Needles	20%		Orange	20%

· · · · · ·

Lavender	30%		Litsea Cubeba	50%
Petitgrain	30%		Ginger	30%
Mandarin	30%		Frankincense	20%
Ginger	10%			

· · · · · ·

Chamomile (Roman)	50%		Spruce	40%
Tangerine	50%		Tangerine	40%
			Fir Needles	20%

MIST SPRAYS

Fill a fine-mist spray bottle with purified water, then add the essential oils. Tighten the cap and shake well. Mist numerous times and breathe in the vapors deeply.

Litsea Cubeba	50 drops		Fir Needles	40 drops
Mandarin	50 drops		Spruce	40 drops
Patchouli	30 drops		Frankincense	40 drops
Ginger	20 drops		Lemon	30 drops
Pure Water	4 ounces		Pure Water	4 ounces

• • • • • •   • • • • • •

Bay	40 drops		Lemon	50 drops
Orange	30 drops		Grapefruit	30 drops
Petitgrain	30 drops		Vetiver	30 drops
Lavender	30 drops		Ginger	30 drops
Peru Balsam	20 drops		Frankincense	10 drops
Pure Water	4 ounces		Pure Water	4 ounces

• • • • • •   • • • • • •

Mandarin	40 drops		Litsea Cubeba	35 drops
Lemon	40 drops		Peru Balsam	35 drops
Frankincense	25 drops		Fir Needles	30 drops
Patchouli	25 drops		Basil (Sweet)	25 drops
Peru Balsam	20 drops		Ginger	25 drops
Pure Water	4 ounces		Pure Water	4 ounces

REFLECTION WORKSHEET*

Insights on direction in life: _____

_____

_____

_____

_____

_____

_____

Planned changes: _____

_____

_____

_____

_____

_____

_____

_____

_____

Actions to be taken: _____

_____

_____

_____

_____

_____

_____

_____

_____

*Please make a copy of this worksheet and fill it out.

VISUALIZATION TO ACHIEVE GOALS

On the Visualization Worksheet, write down a goal you wish to achieve. Make sure it is realistic. List obstacles. Make a plan of action to overcome the obstacles, and list guidelines for measuring your accomplishment. (See Sample Visualization Worksheet, page 55.)

If you've had problems achieving this goal previously and failed, don't give up. There is a very important element called timing. Sometimes the timing is not right. Respect that—but don't allow it to discourage you from attempting the goal again.

- Choose one of these methods: application, diffusor, or mist spray; select and use a formula.
- Do the relaxation exercise on page 24. Then envision yourself in every detail from beginning to finish, accomplishing your goal. See yourself successful.
- Repeat this exercise as often as possible, ideally three to four times a week for about 20–30 minutes each time. The more you practice this exercise, the easier it will become.

For example: If your goal is to lose 15 pounds in three months, write down how you are going to make it happen. Your action plan can involve exercising 30 minutes, three days a week, receiving cellulite treatments, and making healthy dietary changes. Be specific. Once you have completed this step, you are ready to use visualization to reinforce your goal. Visualize yourself acting out your plan of action in full detail within the time you've allotted. Picture yourself losing weight and seeing yourself in the mirror looking and feeling great.

If doubts, contradictory thoughts, or negative feelings present themselves during or after the visualization, allow them to pass on. Do not analyze, suppress, or resist them, since resistance gives them power by diverting away your thoughts. Just return to your positive visions and the doubts and negative feelings will leave of their own accord.

Once you are nearing the attainment of your goal, visualize the action to maintain your achievement. It's great to attain and even greater to maintain! As Henry Ford said, "If you think you can do it or if you think you can't—you're right!"

It's all up to you!

APPLICATION

Apply one of these formulas to the upper chest and back of the neck until the oil is fully absorbed into the skin. Breathe in the vapors deeply.

Myrtle	4 drops	Chamomile (Roman)	4 drops
Cinnamon Leaf	3 drops	Orange	3 drops
Sandalwood	3 drops	Copaiba	2 drops
Carrier Oil	2 teaspoons	Rosemary	1 drop
		Carrier Oil	2 teaspoons

Clary Sage	3 drops
Citronella	3 drops
Helichrysum	2 drops
Rosemary	2 drops
Carrier Oil	2 teaspoons

• • • • • •

Coriander	3 drops
Peru Balsam	3 drops
Basil (Sweet)	3 drops
Copaiba	1 drop
Carrier Oil	2 teaspoons

• • • • • •

Chamomile (Roman)	4 drops
Basil (Sweet)	3 drops
Patchouli	3 drops
Carrier Oil	2 teaspoons

• • • • • •

Petitgrain	3 drops
Chamomile (Roman)	3 drops
Juniper Berry	3 drops
Sandalwood	1 drop
Carrier Oil	2 teaspoons

Helichrysum	4 drops
Cinnamon Leaf	3 drops
Dill	3 drops
Carrier Oil	2 teaspoons

• • • • • •

Clary Sage	3 drops
Patchouli	3 drops
Grapefruit	3 drops
Lemongrass	1 drop
Carrier Oil	2 teaspoons

• • • • • •

Orange	4 drops
Dill	2 drops
Anise	2 drops
Labdanum	2 drops
Carrier Oil	2 teaspoons

• • • • • •

Fennel (Sweet)	3 drops
Grapefruit	3 drops
Cinnamon Leaf	2 drops
Peru Balsam	2 drops
Carrier Oil	2 teaspoons

DIFFUSOR

Depending on the type of diffusor you have, place the essential oils on the diffusor pad or in the glass bottle to disperse the aroma into the air.

Petitgrain	50%
Cinnamon Leaf	40%
Orange	10%

Geranium	30%
Myrtle	30%
Anise	20%
Chamomile (Roman)	20%

Grapefruit	30%		Lavender	40%
Juniper Berry	30%		Clove	20%
Tangerine	20%		Coriander	20%
Rosemary	10%		Palmarosa	20%
Cinnamon Leaf	10%			

MIST SPRAYS

Fill a fine-mist spray bottle with purified water, then add the essential oils. Tighten the cap and shake well. Mist numerous times and breathe in the vapors deeply.

Patchouli	40 drops		Spearmint	40 drops
Geranium	40 drops		Cajeput	40 drops
Elemi	40 drops		Cedarwood (Atlas)	30 drops
Cinnamon Leaf	30 drops		Basil (Sweet)	30 drops
Pure Water	4 ounces		Chamomile (Roman)	10 drops
			Pure Water	4 ounces

• • • • • •

Chamomile (Roman)	50 drops		Lavender	50 drops
Patchouli	50 drops		Cinnamon Leaf	40 drops
Lemongrass	50 drops		Lemon	40 drops
Pure Water	4 ounces		Rosemary	20 drops
			Pure Water	4 ounces

• • • • • •

Copaiba	40 drops		Cinnamon Leaf	30 drops
Cypress	40 drops		Fennel (Sweet)	30 drops
Chamomile (Roman)	40 drops		Coriander	30 drops
Orange	30 drops		Copaiba	30 drops
Pure Water	4 ounces		Mandarin	30 drops
			Pure Water	4 ounces

SAMPLE VISUALIZATION WORKSHEET

Today's date: *January 2*

1. My goal will be achieved by this date: *April 2*

2. My goal is to: *lose 15 pounds in three months*

3. The obstacles/reasons in the past that have prevented me from obtaining long-term
   results are: *I am tempted by the fattening foods my family members
   bring into the house. I lack willpower to abstain from these foods.*

4. I am overcoming these obstacles by specifically taking this/these action(s): *Today
   I am starting the visualization exercises to strengthen my willpower.*

5. Action plan: *A. Visualization exercises at least 4X weekly*
   B. Exercise workout—30 minutes, 3X weekly
   C. Cellulite treatments, at least 3X monthly
   D. Dietary changes (see Chapter 8, "Shaping Up")
   E. Other (activities you enjoy to feel good about yourself)
   F. Introspection exercises monthly to measure progress

6. I will examine and measure my progress in these ways:
   A. How I feel about myself
   B. How much weight I have lost

VISUALIZATION WORKSHEET*

Today's date:_____

1. My goal will be achieved by this date: _____

2. My goal is to:_____

_____

3. The obstacles/reasons in the past that have prevented me from obtaining long-term results are: _____

_____

_____

4. I am overcoming these obstacles by specifically taking this/these action(s):

_____

_____

5. Action plan: _____

_____

_____

_____

_____

_____

6. I will examine and measure my progress in these ways: _____

_____

_____

_____

Please make a copy of this sheet and fill it out.

CHAPTER 5

THE NEED FOR TOUCH

❁ ❁ ❁

A LOVER'S CARESS, friends comforting each other with a hug, a mother's warm embrace—touch is the most powerful form of communication. In human relationships, words only account for about 10 percent of all expression, the remainder is comprised of body language, gestures, and touch. Touch is the first sense to function in humans. It is operative even before the higher brain centers begin to work.

The skin contains millions of nerve endings; when touched, they send messages to the brain, stimulating various organs and glands to secrete chemicals and hormones that affect the body. The brain's perception of the type of touch determines the body's reaction. If the touch is not of a threatening nature, the body's response will be favorable. Even comatose patients show higher hemoglobin counts after being touched.

Many people are surprised to learn that lack of touch can impair growth in children. It is known that the growth hormone ACTH, which is produced by the pituitary gland, is insufficiently secreted by certain children who live in an atmosphere deprived of tactile stimulation. When these youngsters are transferred to an environment where they receive touch, hormone secretions return to a normal level.

Throughout the 19th century, large numbers of children raised in orphanages, devoid of touch, died from a disease called "wasting away." As late as the 1920s the death rate for infants under one year of age, in orphanages throughout the United States, was over 60%.

Touch is also extremely vital to animals. Newborn animals rely on their mother's touch, otherwise they will die within the first few hours after birth. Dairy farmers report that hand-milked cows give richer and larger amounts of milk than cows milked by machine.

Regardless of age, everyone needs to give and receive touch. Without its warmth to reassure and soothe us, we are denying ourselves perhaps one of our most vital and basic needs.

FORMULAS

MASSAGE

Massage is the oldest form of therapy to help soothe and provide comfort to a tense body. Massage works by releasing tight muscles and stimulating the nerves, blood circulation, and lymphatic system to eliminate toxins. Not only enjoyable, massage can assist in bringing people closer to one another.

CHILDREN SIX MONTHS TO ONE YEAR OLD

Mix ingredients together and use the amount necessary. Massage on the back of the neck, shoulders, and back, until the oil is absorbed into the skin. After the massage, dab on some cornstarch to dry the area. Save the remaining oil for the next time.

Take precautions so children do not get oil on their hands and then touch or rub their eyes.

Lavender	3 drops		Sandalwood	3 drops
Mandarin	2 drops		Chamomile (Roman)	2 drops
Hazelnut	2 tablespoons		Hazelnut	2 tablespoons
• • • • • •			• • • • • •	
Grapefruit	3 drops		Orange	3 drops
Lavender	2 drops		Ylang-Ylang	2 drops
Hazelnut	2 tablespoons		Hazelnut	2 tablespoons

CHILDREN ONE TO FIVE YEARS OLD

As the child grows, additional essential oils can be used and the amount of drops increased.

Mix all ingredients together and use the amount necessary. Massage the formula on the back of the neck, shoulders, and back, until the oil is fully absorbed into the skin. After the massage, dab on some cornstarch to dry the area. Save the remaining oil for the next time.

Take precautions so children do not get oil on their hands and then touch or rub their eyes.

These formulas will bring on a happy and peaceful state.

Geranium	3 drops		Lavender	3 drops
Sandalwood	2 drops		Spruce	2 drops
Hazelnut	1 tablespoon		Hazelnut	1 tablespoon
• • • • • •			• • • • • •	
Mandarin	3 drops		Ylang-Ylang	3 drops
Copaiba	2 drops		Bois de Rose	2 drops
Hazelnut	1 tablespoon		Hazelnut	1 tablespoon

CHILDREN FIVE TO FIFTEEN YEARS OLD

Massage one of the formulas on the back of the neck, shoulders, back, and the upper chest, until the oil is fully absorbed into the skin. After the massage, dab on some cornstarch to dry the area. Take precautions so children do not get oil on their hands and then touch or rub their eyes.

CALMING

Tangerine	4 drops	Orange	4 drops
Marjoram	3 drops	Vetiver	3 drops
Carrier Oil	1 tablespoon	Carrier Oil	1 tablespoon
• • • • • •		• • • • • •	
Sandalwood	4 drops	Marjoram	4 drops
Petitgrain	3 drops	Copaiba	3 drops
Carrier Oil	1 tablespoon	Carrier Oil	1 tablespoon

REFRESHING

Spearmint	5 drops	Peppermint	5 drops
Sandalwood	2 drops	Bergamot	2 drops
Carrier Oil	1 tablespoon	Carrier Oil	1 tablespoon
• • • • • •		• • • • • •	
Lime	4 drops	Lemon	4 drops
Eucalyptus	3 drops	Tea Tree	3 drops
Carrier Oil	1 tablespoon	Carrier Oil	1 tablespoon

FOR LOVERS

Spend an enjoyable evening together by giving each other a sensual massage. Massage the formula on the back of the neck, shoulders, down the back, chest, and abdominal area until the oil is absorbed into the skin. For best results, massage for 30 minutes.

Patchouli	6 drops	Sandalwood	6 drops
Spruce	5 drops	Vanilla	5 drops
Sandalwood	5 drops	Pepper (Black)	5 drops
Vanilla	4 drops	Bay	4 drops
Carrier Oil	4 teaspoons	Carrier Oil	4 teaspoons

Tangerine	6 drops		Orange	5 drops
Spruce	5 drops		Patchouli	5 drops
Ylang-Ylang	5 drops		Nutmeg	5 drops
Ginger	4 drops		Ylang-Ylang	5 drops
Carrier Oil	4 teaspoons		Carrier Oil	4 teaspoons

• • • • • •   • • • • • •

Vanilla	5 drops		Peru Balsam	5 drops
Helichrysum	5 drops		Orange	5 drops
Clary Sage	5 drops		Palmarosa	5 drops
Litsea Cubeba	5 drops		Neroli	5 drops
Carrier Oil	4 teaspoons		Carrier Oil	4 teaspoons

• • • • • •   • • • • • •

Peru Balsam	5 drops		Sandalwood	5 drops
Neroli	4 drops		Mandarin	4 drops
Bois de Rose	4 drops		Cinnamon Leaf	4 drops
Spikenard	4 drops		Vanilla	4 drops
Cinnamon Leaf	3 drops		Cumin	3 drops
Carrier Oil	4 teaspoons		Carrier Oil	4 teaspoons

MOOD UPLIFTING

Massage one of these formulas on the upper chest, back of the neck, shoulders, and down the back until the oil is fully absorbed into the skin. Breathe in the vapors deeply. For best results, massage for 30 minutes.

Peppermint	8 drops		Geranium	5 drops
Copaiba	5 drops		Tangerine	5 drops
Lemon	4 drops		Vetiver	5 drops
Thyme	3 drops		Citronella	5 drops
Carrier Oil	4 teaspoons		Carrier Oil	4 teaspoons

• • • • • •   • • • • • •

Bois de Rose	6 drops		Frankincense	5 drops
Ylang-Ylang	5 drops		Mandarin	5 drops
Benzoin	5 drops		Cypress	5 drops
Basil (Sweet)	4 drops		Bay	5 drops
Carrier Oil	4 teaspoons		Carrier Oil	4 teaspoons

Peru Balsam	6 drops	Petitgrain	5 drops
Bay	5 drops	Bergamot	5 drops
Bergamot	5 drops	Geranium	5 drops
Basil (Sweet)	4 drops	Labdanum	5 drops
Carrier Oil	4 teaspoons	Carrier Oil	4 teaspoons

• • • • • • • • • • • •

Mandarin	4 drops	Hyssop Decumbens	5 drops
Spearmint	4 drops	Palmarosa	4 drops
Grapefruit	4 drops	Petitgrain	4 drops
Frankincense	4 drops	Vanilla	4 drops
Spikenard	4 drops	Chamomile (Roman)	3 drops
Carrier Oil	4 teaspoons	Carrier Oil	4 teaspoons

RELAXING

Massage one of these formulas on the upper chest, back of the neck, shoulders, down the back, and the bottoms of the feet until the oil is fully absorbed into the skin. Breathe in the vapors deeply. For best results, massage for 30 minutes.

Celery	5 drops	Vetiver	5 drops
Orange	5 drops	Elemi	5 drops
Frankincense	5 drops	Marjoram	4 drops
Copaiba	5 drops	Lavender	4 drops
Carrier Oil	4 teaspoons	Cedarwood (Atlas)	2 drops
		Carrier Oil	4 teaspoons

• • • • • • • • • • • •

Orange	5 drops	Lemongrass	5 drops
Labdanum	4 drops	Mandarin	5 drops
Copaiba	4 drops	Sandalwood	4 drops
Basil (Sweet)	4 drops	Petitgrain	4 drops
Chamomile (Roman)	3 drops	Elemi	2 drops
Carrier Oil	4 teaspoons	Carrier Oil	4 teaspoons

Spikenard	4 drops		Bois de Rose	5 drops
Celery	4 drops		Litsea Cubeba	4 drops
Neroli	4 drops		Chamomile (Roman)	4 drops
Mandarin	4 drops		Ylang-Ylang	4 drops
Peru Balsam	4 drops		Clary Sage	3 drops
Carrier Oil	4 teaspoons		Carrier Oil	4 teaspoons

CHAPTER 6

CARING FOR YOUR BODY

❂ ❂ ❂

SKIN

OUR REMARKABLE SKIN—perhaps the most resilient organ of the body. An extraordinary protector and our first line of defense against the assault of the outside world, it can endure harsh weather and environmental conditions, yet can be sensitive and gentle enough to respond to a kind and loving touch.

Covering every inch of our outer body, the skin also performs many other vital functions. Operating as a thermostat, it helps regulate body temperature by conveying signals to the brain via nerve cells. And when healthy, the skin helps the body eliminate about 25% of its waste through perspiration.

Often referred to as a mirror of health, the skin is a reflection of the inner condition of the body, and the showcase to the world. Closely related to our emotions, it turns pale when we are ill or stressed and is radiant and glowing when we are healthy and happy. Fortunately for us, the skin continually replenishes itself, creating millions of new cells each day.

From our early formation to the end of our life, our skin is always there to protect us.

HAIR

One of the first things we notice when we look at a person is the person's hair. Hair not only accentuates the appearance, it insulates the head from temperature variances; acts as a cushion to protect the skull; allows sweat to evaporate; and also acts as a sensor when touched.

Each hair grows inside a tube-like follicle and at the base of each follicle is a hair bulb. This bulb is full of blood vessels that deliver oxygen and nourishment to the root. The cells inside the bulb are alive. As they die, they are pushed upward to form the visible hair on the head.

Since the hair's appearance is determined by the condition of health inside the hair bulbs, the nutritional intake, circulatory system, and care of the scalp play important roles. Under the scalp are blood vessels, nerves endings, sebaceous glands, sweat glands, and the subcutaneous layer of fat cells. The sebaceous glands surround about half of each hair follicle. Their purpose is to lubricate the hair and scalp with an oily secretion called sebum. The sebaceous glands become more active during times of stress, physical activity, or alcohol consumption.

FORMULAS

BATHS

Besides being necessary for hygiene, baths are beneficial for good health. These formulas will help moisturize and scent the skin.

    Fill the bathtub with water as warm as you like. Add the formula, dispersing it evenly throughout the water. Enter the bath immediately, since the essential oils evaporate quickly. Relax and enjoy your bath for 30 minutes.

Lavender	5 drops		Palmarosa	5 drops
Bois de Rose	5 drops		Mandarin	5 drops
Vanilla	5 drops		Cedarwood (Atlas)	5 drops
Carrier Oil	1 teaspoon		Carrier Oil	1 teaspoon

• • • • • • •

Copaiba	6 drops		Bois de Rose	7 drops
Sandalwood	5 drops		Patchouli	4 drops
Geranium	4 drops		Litsea Cubeba	4 drops
Carrier Oil	1 teaspoon		Carrier Oil	1 teaspoon

• • • • • • •

Sandalwood	7 drops		Guaiacwood	5 drops
Mandarin	5 drops		Tangerine	5 drops
Frankincense	3 drops		Copaiba	5 drops
Carrier Oil	1 teaspoon		Carrier Oil	1 teaspoon

CHAPPED LIPS

These formulas should be very helpful to moisturize chapped lips. Heat a small pot of water, place the shea butter into a small, wide-mouthed glass jar, and put the jar into the pot of water. When the shea butter is melted, add the carrier oil, mix well, and remove from the heat. As the mixture cools, add the essential oils and stir well. Apply the creme several times daily as needed.

Lavender	20 drops		Frankincense	10 drops
Bois de Rose	5 drops		Geranium	10 drops
Shea Butter	6 teaspoons		Palmarosa	5 drops
Sesame	3 teaspoons		Shea Butter	6 teaspoons
			Sesame	3 teaspoons

Lavender	15 drops		Bois de Rose	12 drops
Patchouli	5 drops		Peru Balsam	8 drops
Frankincense	5 drops		Palmarosa	5 drops
Shea Butter	6 teaspoons		Shea Butter	6 teaspoons
Sesame	3 teaspoons		Sesame	3 teaspoons

• • • • • • •

Copaiba	15 drops		Sandalwood	15 drops
Lavender	10 drops		Elemi	10 drops
Shea Butter	6 teaspoons		Shea Butter	6 teaspoons
Sesame	3 teaspoons		Sesame	3 teaspoons

• • • • • • •

Rose	10 drops		Copaiba	10 drops
Sandalwood	10 drops		Geranium	10 drops
Myrrh	5 drops		Patchouli	5 drops
Shea Butter	6 teaspoons		Shea Butter	6 teaspoons
Sesame	3 teaspoons		Sesame	3 teaspoons

DEODORANTS

These formulas will keep you smelling nice. Apply 10 drops of aloe vera onto each underarm, then combine the formula and rub in well. Finish by patting on cornstarch to dry any remaining residue. Make sure to remove any excess oil with a tissue to prevent clothing from becoming stained. After a woman shaves her underarms it is advisable to wait 15 minutes before applying the deodorant in order to avoid any burning sensation.

Chamomile (Roman)	2 drops		Spikenard	2 drops
Vanilla	2 drops		Lavender	2 drops
Spikenard	2 drops		Vanilla	2 drops

FACIAL SAUNA

These formulas are beneficial to increase circulation to skin cells.

Heat a small pot of water and then pour it into a bowl. Add the essential oils, drape a towel over your head, lean forward, and close your eyes. Allow the vapors to come in contact with your face.

Frankincense	5 drops		Copaiba	6 drops
Lemon	5 drops		Tangerine	4 drops
• • • • • •			• • • • • •	
Bois de Rose	5 drops		Lavender	6 drops
Grapefruit	5 drops		Tea Tree	3 drops
			Peppermint	1 drop
• • • • • •			• • • • • •	
Elemi	6 drops		Sandalwood	5 drops
Lime	4 drops		Tangerine	5 drops

HAIR CARE CREMES

To prepare the formula, place the shea butter into a small wide-mouthed glass jar. Put the jar into the pot of water, and heat on a low flame. When the shea butter is melted, add the carrier oil, mix well, and remove from the heat. As the mixture cools, add the essential oils and stir well.

Rub in aloe vera juice and a small portion of the formula into the scalp once a day.

Cedarwood (Atlas)	20 drops		Sandalwood	20 drops
Bay	10 drops		Bois de Rose	20 drops
Litsea Cubeba	10 drops		Shea Butter	2 tablespoons
Shea Butter	2 tablespoons		Jojoba	8 teaspoons
Jojoba	8 teaspoons			
• • • • • •			• • • • • •	
Elemi	20 drops		Cedarwood (Atlas)	20 drops
Lemon	12 drops		Myrrh	10 drops
Patchouli	8 drops		Spearmint	10 drops
Shea Butter	2 tablespoons		Shea Butter	2 tablespoons
Jojoba	8 teaspoons		Jojoba	8 teaspoons

Myrrh	15 drops	Lavender	20 drops
Copaiba	13 drops	Cedarwood (Atlas)	20 drops
Litsea Cubeba	12 drops	Shea Butter	2 tablespoons
Shea Butter	2 tablespoons	Jojoba	8 teaspoons
Jojoba	8 teaspoons		

• • • • • •   • • • • • •

Ylang-Ylang	15 drops	Rosemary	15 drops
Copaiba	15 drops	Lavender	15 drops
Frankincense	10 drops	Myrrh	10 drops
Shea Butter	2 tablespoons	Shea Butter	2 tablespoons
Jojoba	8 teaspoons	Jojoba	8 teaspoons

• • • • • •   • • • • • •

Ylang-Ylang	17 drops	Sandalwood	20 drops
Lemon	17 drops	Palmarosa	13 drops
Ginger	6 drops	Mandarin	7 drops
Shea Butter	2 tablespoons	Shea Butter	2 tablespoons
Jojoba	8 teaspoons	Jojoba	8 teaspoons

JOCK- AND JANE-ITCH POWDERS

Pour four ounces of cornstarch into a wide-mouthed glass jar, add the essential oils, and mix well. Cap the jar and let sit for several hours before using. Then apply the powder at least once a day until the itching is gone.

Patchouli	40 drops	Litsea Cubeba	50 drops
Lime	40 drops	Cypress	40 drops
Lavender	40 drops	Tea Tree	30 drops
Cornstarch	4 ounces	Cornstarch	4 ounces

• • • • • •   • • • • • •

Lavender	60 drops	Litsea Cubeba	60 drops
Sage	30 drops	Copaiba	40 drops
Cinnamon Leaf	30 drops	Thyme	20 drops
Cornstarch	4 ounces	Cornstarch	4 ounces

Eucalyptus	40 drops		Cedarwood (Atlas)	50 drops
Pine	40 drops		Tangerine	40 drops
Sandalwood	40 drops		Myrtle	30 drops
Cornstarch	4 ounces		Cornstarch	4 ounces

• • • • • •   • • • • • •

Lemon	60 drops		Lavender	60 drops
Patchouli	40 drops		Sandalwood	60 drops
Tea Tree	20 drops		Cornstarch	4 ounces
Cornstarch	4 ounces			

MOUTHWASH

For fresh breath, use one of these formulas. Pour the water in a glass, stir in the essential oils, honey, a pinch of unrefined sea salt (optional), and rinse your mouth. Cap the unused portion and store for later use.

Clove	3 drops		Spearmint	3 drops
Orange	3 drops		Lemon	3 drops
Honey	1 teaspoon		Honey	1 teaspoon
Sea Salt	1 pinch		Sea Salt	1 pinch
Pure Water	4 ounces		Pure Water	4 ounces

• • • • • •   • • • • • •

Anise	3 drops		Cypress	2 drops
Orange	3 drops		Myrrh	2 drops
Honey	1 teaspoon		Mandarin	2 drops
Sea Salt	1 pinch		Honey	1 teaspoon
Pure Water	4 ounces		Sea Salt	1 pinch
			Pure Water	4 ounces

• • • • • •   • • • • • •

Sandalwood	3 drops		Lime	2 drops
Spearmint	3 drops		Tangerine	2 drops
Honey	1 teaspoon		Cypress	2 drops
Sea Salt	1 pinch		Honey	1 teaspoon
Pure Water	4 ounces		Sea Salt	1 pinch
			Pure Water	4 ounces

Sandalwood	4 drops	Cinnamon Leaf	2 drops
Sage	2 drops	Ginger	2 drops
Honey	1 teaspoon	Orange	2 drops
Sea Salt	1 pinch	Honey	1 teaspoon
Pure Water	4 ounces	Sea Salt	1 pinch
		Pure Water	4 ounces

PRE-ELECTRIC SHAVING POWDERS

Pour four ounces of cornstarch into a wide-mouthed glass jar. Stir the essential oils in well, cap the jar, and let sit for several hours before using. Apply the powder to the area before shaving.

Myrrh	45 drops	Juniper Berry	30 drops
Tangerine	45 drops	Lemon	30 drops
Cornstarch	4 ounces	Fir Needles	30 drops
		Cornstarch	4 ounces

• • • • • •

Cypress	45 drops	Ylang-Ylang	50 drops
Orange	45 drops	Citronella	20 drops
Cornstarch	4 ounces	Myrrh	20 drops
		Cornstarch	4 ounces

• • • • • •

Litsea Cubeba	40 drops	Lavender	45 drops
Bois de Rose	30 drops	Tangerine	45 drops
Patchouli	20 drops	Cornstarch	4 ounces
Cornstarch	4 ounces		

• • • • • •

Sandalwood	60 drops	Peppermint	45 drops
Spearmint	30 drops	Copaiba	45 drops
Cornstarch	4 ounces	Cornstarch	4 ounces

• • • • • •

Lemon	60 drops	Sandalwood	40 drops
Cypress	20 drops	Myrtle	25 drops
Copaiba	10 drops	Grapefruit	25 drops
Cornstarch	4 ounces	Cornstarch	4 ounces

Spruce	30 drops		Litsea Cubeba	50 drops
Pine	30 drops		Cedarwood (Atlas)	40 drops
Cedarwood (Atlas)	30 drops		Cornstarch	4 ounces
Cornstarch	4 ounces			

SHAVING CREMES

To prepare, place the shea butter into a small wide-mouthed glass jar. Put the jar into a small pot of water, and heat on a low flame. When the butter is melted, add the carrier oil, mix well, and remove from the heat. As the mixture cools add the essential oils and stir well.

Apply a small amount to the skin, rub in, and shave.

Sandalwood	10 drops		Copaiba	10 drops
Litsea Cubeba	10 drops		Peppermint	10 drops
Shea Butter	2 tablespoons		Shea Butter	2 tablespoons
Carrier Oil	3 tablespoons		Carrier Oil	3 tablespoons

• • • • • •

Fir Needles	5 drops		Cypress	8 drops
Spearmint	5 drops		Grapefruit	7 drops
Cedarwood (Atlas)	5 drops		Neroli	5 drops
Pine	5 drops		Shea Butter	2 tablespoons
Shea Butter	2 tablespoons		Carrier Oil	3 tablespoons
Carrier Oil	3 tablespoons			

• • • • • •

Bois de Rose	7 drops		Spruce	13 drops
Litsea Cubeba	7 drops		Coriander	7 drops
Patchouli	6 drops		Shea Butter	2 tablespoons
Shea Butter	2 tablespoons		Carrier Oil	3 tablespoons
Carrier Oil	3 tablespoons			

• • • • • •

Bois de Rose	10 drops		Geranium	7 drops
Lavender	10 drops		Cardamom	7 drops
Shea Butter	2 tablespoons		Myrtle	6 drops
Carrier Oil	3 tablespoons		Shea Butter	2 tablespoons
			Carrier Oil	3 tablespoons

Rose	7 drops	Sandalwood	10 drops
Palmarosa	7 drops	Tangerine	7 drops
Bois de Rose	6 drops	Fir Needles	3 drops
Shea Butter	2 tablespoons	Shea Butter	2 tablespoons
Carrier Oil	3 tablespoons	Carrier Oil	3 tablespoons

SKIN CARE CREMES

The skin gets taken for granted due to its ability to recover from burns, bruises, cuts, scrapes, scratches, along with other types of injuries and wounds that are inflicted in the course of our daily life.

Apply a small amount of one of these formulas daily to help keep your skin looking younger, healthier, and feeling softer.

To prepare the formula, place the shea butter into a small wide-mouthed glass jar. Put the jar into a small pot of water, and heat on a low flame. When the butter is melted, add the carrier oil, mix well, and remove from the heat. As the mixture cools, add the essential oils, and stir well.

Frankincense	20 drops	Lavender	20 drops
Myrrh	8 drops	Rose	15 drops
Litsea Cubeba	7 drops	Shea Butter	2 tablespoons
Shea Butter	2 tablepoons	Sesame	8 teaspoons
Sesame	8 teaspoons		

• • • • • •

Ylang-Ylang	15 drops	Copaiba	15 drops
Myrrh	12 drops	Myrrh	11 drops
Orange	8 drops	Peppermint	9 drops
Shea Butter	2 tablespoons	Shea Butter	2 tablespoons
Sesame	8 teaspoons	Sesame	8 teaspoons

• • • • • •

Peru Balsam	20 drops	Sandalwood	15 drops
Peppermint	15 drops	Bois de Rose	10 drops
Shea Butter	2 tablespoons	Helichrysum	10 drops
Sesame	8 teaspoons	Shea Butter	2 tablespoons
		Sesame	8 teaspoons

Frankincense	12 drops		Ylang-Ylang	15 drops
Lemon	12 drops		Copaiba	10 drops
Patchouli	11 drops		Citronella	10 drops
Shea Butter	2 tablespoons		Shea Butter	2 tablespoons
Sesame	8 teaspoons		Sesame	8 teaspoons

• • • • • •   • • • • • •

Rosemary	15 drops		Spearmint	12 drops
Elemi	10 drops		Geranium	12 drops
Bois de Rose	10 drops		Sandalwood	11 drops
Shea Butter	2 tablespoons		Shea Butter	2 tablespoons
Sesame	8 teaspoons		Sesame	8 teaspoons

CHAPTER 7

SURRENDER YOUR STRESS

❁ ❁ ❁

STRESS IS THE BODY'S response when life's demands become overwhelming. It is especially produced on occasions when we suppress our natural instincts or withhold our feelings. If the stressed state is allowed to linger, it causes considerable damage to the body. The adrenal glands can become exhausted, resulting in impaired physical and mental functioning, reduced energy levels, fatigue, and depression. It may be responsible for an increase in blood pressure, immune-system suppression, heart disease, and other organ and nervous system disorders.

One of the great paradoxes is that with the advancement of modern technology—intended to make life easier and improved—stress-related illnesses are increasingly rising. It has been estimated that as many as 75% of all medical complaints are stress related.

DEEP BREATHING

Breathing is the foundation of life. However, in most large cities the air pollution from industry and vehicle emissions is so great that it discourages people from breathing deeply. In addition, stress has the same effect, causing a person to breathe shallowly. Deep breathing is essential to relieve stress and maintain good health and well-being. By using essential oils and practicing deep breathing exercises daily, you should notice favorable results.

SLEEP

High levels of stress and the inability to achieve a restful sleep cause a vicious cycle. If you are highly stressed it is difficult to get a good night's rest—and if you don't get a good night's rest, you're likely to develop more stress.

According to estimates, about 17% of the population has difficulty sleeping. Some have problems falling asleep and others wake up and have difficulty returning to sleep.

HELPFUL TIPS FOR BETTER SLEEP

* Don't eat for at least three hours before bedtime.
* Avoid excitement before going to sleep.
* Make sure your bedroom is clean and neat.
* Use natural fibres for bed linens, covers, and night wear.
* Do deep breathing exercises using essential oils.
* Receive a relaxing massage with essential oils before going to bed.

FORMULAS

CANDLELIGHT DINNER

AROMA LAMP

Place an aroma lamp or a small electric potpourri pot in the center of the table. When dinner is served, fill the container with water, add the essential oils, and heat. Play soft music, light the candles, dim the lights, and enjoy a candlelight dinner.

FLORAL

Ylang-Ylang	8 drops	Rose	7 drops
Tangerine	5 drops	Peru Balsam	6 drops
Sandalwood	4 drops	Clove	4 drops
Cumin	3 drops	Pepper (Black)	3 drops
• • • • • •		• • • • • •	
Vanilla	5 drops	Bergamot	8 drops
Neroli	5 drops	Hyssop Decumbens	7 drops
Orange	5 drops	Neroli	5 drops
Sandalwood	5 drops		

MINTY

Spearmint	9 drops	Peppermint	9 drops
Fennel (Sweet)	4 drops	Sandalwood	6 drops
Patchouli	4 drops	Anise	5 drops
Allspice	3 drops		

Peppermint	10 drops	Spearmint	9 drops
Spruce	6 drops	Eucalyptus	5 drops
Cedarwood (Atlas)	4 drops	Sandalwood	4 drops
		Allspice	2 drops

CITRUS

Lemongrass	8 drops	Orange	8 drops
Palmarosa	4 drops	Peru Balsam	8 drops
Ginger	4 drops	Petitgrain	4 drops
Patchouli	4 drops		

• • • • • •

Grapefruit	6 drops	Lemon	6 drops
Sandalwood	6 drops	Mandarin	5 drops
Litsea Cubeba	5 drops	Cardamom	5 drops
Spruce	4 drops	Cedarwood (Atlas)	4 drops

FOREST

Spruce	5 drops	Fir Needles	5 drops
Eucalyptus	4 drops	Rosemary	5 drops
Fir Needles	4 drops	Cedarwood (Atlas)	4 drops
Sandalwood	4 drops	Frankincense	3 drops
Peppermint	3 drops	Allspice	3 drops

• • • • • •

Sandalwood	5 drops	Spruce	9 drops
Spruce	4 drops	Cedarwood (Atlas)	5 drops
Pine	4 drops	Peru Balsam	3 drops
Cajeput	4 drops	Anise	3 drops
Myrtle	3 drops		

DEEP BREATHING

APPLICATION

Apply one of these formulas to the upper chest and abdomen, until the oil is fully absorbed into the skin. Breathe in the vapors deeply.

Eucalyptus	4 drops		Fir Needles	4 drops
Peppermint	4 drops		Cajeput	4 drops
Sandalwood	2 drops		Cedarwood (Atlas)	2 drops
Carrier Oil	1 teaspoon		Carrier Oil	1 teaspoon

• • • • • •   • • • • • •

Tea Tree	4 drops		Copaiba	4 drops
Spearmint	4 drops		Grapefruit	3 drops
Copaiba	2 drops		Anise	3 drops
Carrier Oil	1 teaspoon		Carrier Oil	1 teaspoon

• • • • • •   • • • • • •

Myrtle	4 drops		Sandalwood	3 drops
Eucalyptus	4 drops		Frankincense	3 drops
Cedarwood (Atlas)	2 drops		Spruce	3 drops
Carrier Oil	1 teaspoon		Peppermint	1 drop
			Carrier Oil	1 teaspoon

• • • • • •   • • • • • •

Lavender	4 drops		Hyssop Decumbens	5 drops
Sandalwood	3 drops		Tea Tree	4 drops
Marjoram	2 drops		Cedarwood (Atlas)	2 drops
Spearmint	1 drop		Carrier Oil	1 teaspoon
Carrier Oil	1 teaspoon			

DIFFUSOR

Depending on the type of diffusor you have, place the essential oils on the diffusor pad or in the glass bottle to disperse the aroma into the air.

Hyssop Decumbens	50%		Lavender	40%
Frankincense	50%		Eucalyptus	30%
			Hyssop Decumbens	30%

Fir Needles	50%		Cypress	25%
Tea Tree	20%		Spearmint	25%
Eucalyptus	20%		Cajeput	25%
Juniper Berry	10%		Lemon	25%

• • • • • •   • • • • • •

Peppermint	30%		Myrtle	30%
Tea Tree	25%		Lime	30%
Lavender	25%		Cubeb	20%
Spruce	20%		Fir Needles	20%

MIST SPRAYS

Fill a fine-mist spray bottle with purified water, then add the essential oils. Tighten the cap and shake well. Mist numerous times and breathe in the vapors deeply.

Lavender	50 drops		Copaiba	50 drops
Cedarwood (Atlas)	50 drops		Eucalyptus	30 drops
Spearmint	50 drops		Peppermint	30 drops
Pure Water	4 ounces		Petitgrain	30 drops
			Clove	10 drops
			Pure Water	4 ounces

• • • • • •   • • • • • •

Cajeput	40 drops		Petitgrain	30 drops
Juniper Berry	25 drops		Myrtle	30 drops
Rosemary	25 drops		Spruce	30 drops
Tea Tree	25 drops		Frankincense	30 drops
Spearmint	25 drops		Cubeb	30 drops
Copaiba	10 drops		Pure Water	4 ounces
Pure Water	4 ounces			

• • • • • •   • • • • • •

Lavender	50 drops		Frankincense	50 drops
Helichrysum	50 drops		Hyssop Decumbens	50 drops
Hyssop Decumbens	50 drops		Lemon	50 drops
Pure Water	4 ounces		Pure Water	4 ounces

SLEEP PEACEFULLY

APPLICATION

Apply one of these formulas to the upper chest and back of the neck until the oil is fully absorbed into the skin. Breathe in the vapors deeply.

Marjoram	4 drops	Benzoin	4 drops
Basil (Sweet)	3 drops	Marjoram	3 drops
Vetiver	3 drops	Petitgrain	3 drops
Carrier Oil	2 teaspoons	Carrier Oil	2 teaspoons
• • • • • •		• • • • • •	
Peru Balsam	4 drops	Cedarwood (Atlas)	3 drops
Orange	3 drops	Neroli	3 drops
Basil (Sweet)	3 drops	Litsea Cubeba	2 drops
Carrier Oil	2 teaspoons	Vetiver	2 drops
• • • • • •		Carrier Oil	2 teaspoons
		• • • • • •	
Sea Buckthorn	5 drops	Spikenard	5 drops
Neroli	3 drops	Sea Buckthorn	5 drops
Mandarin	2 drops	Carrier Oil	1 teaspoon
Carrier Oil	1 teaspoon	• • • • • •	
• • • • • •			
Chamomile (Roman)	4 drops	Chamomile (Roman)	5 drops
Myrtle	2 drops	Lavender	5 drops
Oregano	2 drops	Carrier Oil	2 teaspoons
Tangerine	2 drops		
Carrier Oil	2 teaspoons		

DIFFUSOR

Depending on the type of diffusor you have, place the essential oils on the diffusor pad or in the glass bottle to disperse the aroma into the air.

Petitgrain	50%	Chamomile (Roman)	25%
Orange	20%	Dill	25%
Ylang-Ylang	15%	Petitgrain	25%
Marjoram	15%	Basil (Sweet)	25%

Marjoram	50%	Tangerine	50%
Petitgrain	30%	Marjoram	30%
Lavender	20%	Basil (Sweet)	10%
		Allspice	10%

MIST SPRAYS

Fill a fine-mist spray bottle with purified water, then add the essential oils. Tighten the cap and shake well. Mist numerous times and breathe in the vapors deeply.

Marjoram	75 drops	Vetiver	75 drops
Tangerine	40 drops	Chamomile (Roman)	40 drops
Copaiba	35 drops	Litsea Cubeba	35 drops
Pure Water	4 ounces	Pure Water	4 ounces

• • • • • •　　　　　　• • • • • •

Petitgrain	60 drops	Lavender	50 drops
Basil (Sweet)	40 drops	Celery	40 drops
Cedarwood (Atlas)	40 drops	Lemongrass	40 drops
Anise	10 drops	Copaiba	20 drops
Pure Water	4 ounces	Pure Water	4 ounces

STOP SNORING!

Snoring can cause stress to other people in the house who are kept awake by the noisy snorer. Many married couples have to sleep in separate rooms because one spouse snores. These formulas should help if used over a period of time.

DIFFUSOR

Depending on the type of diffusor you have, place the essential oils on the diffusor pad or in the glass bottle to disperse the aroma into the air.

Bois de Rose	25%	Cajeput	20%
Lavender	25%	Thyme	20%
Cajeput	25%	Anise	20%
Cubeb	15%	Lavender	20%
Eucalyptus	10%	Juniper Berry	20%

Lavender	40%		Marjoram	50%
Petitgrain	35%		Myrtle	25%
Thyme	25%		Litsea Cubeba	25%

· · · · · · ·   · · · · · ·

Lavender	50%		Spruce	50%
Allspice	25%		Marjoram	25%
Petitgrain	25%		Lavender	25%

MASSAGE

Massage on the upper chest, abdomen, back of the neck, and shoulders until the oil is absorbed into the skin. Breathe in the vapors deeply. For best results, massage for 30 minutes.

Lavender	6 drops		Cedarwood (Atlas)	7 drops
Sandalwood	6 drops		Marjoram	6 drops
Copaiba	4 drops		Myrtle	4 drops
Myrtle	4 drops		Peru Balsam	3 drops
Sesame	4 teaspoons		Sesame	4 teaspoons

· · · · · · ·   · · · · · ·

Peru Balsam	8 drops		Cedarwood (Atlas)	7 drops
Marjoram	6 drops		Labdanum	7 drops
Pepper (Black)	3 drops		Basil (Sweet)	3 drops
Cajeput	3 drops		Petitgrain	3 drops
Sesame	4 teaspoons		Sesame	4 teaspoons

· · · · · · ·   · · · · · ·

Sandalwood	6 drops		Cedarwood (Atlas)	6 drops
Grapefruit	5 drops		Lavender	6 drops
Lavender	5 drops		Bois de Rose	4 drops
Lemongrass	4 drops		Frankincense	4 drops
Sesame	4 teaspoons		Sesame	4 teaspoons

· · · · · · ·   · · · · · ·

Peru Balsam	7 drops		Sandalwood	7 drops
Bois de Rose	5 drops		Chamomile (Roman)	7 drops
Copaiba	4 drops		Marjoram	4 drops
Myrtle	4 drops		Thyme	2 drops
Sesame	4 teaspoons		Sesame	4 teaspoons

MIST SPRAYS

Fill a fine-mist spray bottle with water, then add essential oils. Tighten the cap and shake well. Before bedtime, mist numerous times over the snorer's head and have him/her inhale the vapors deeply. If the person begins to snore during the night, mist the spray again.

Lavender	50 drops		Marjoram	60 drops
Cedarwood (Atlas)	40 drops		Sandalwood	50 drops
Copaiba	30 drops		Bois de Rose	20 drops
Juniper Berry	30 drops		Litsea Cubeba	20 drops
Pure Water	4 ounces		Pure Water	4 ounces

• • • • • •   • • • • • •

Cedarwood (Atlas)	60 drops		Cedarwood (Atlas)	50 drops
Myrtle	50 drops		Litsea Cubeba	35 drops
Spruce	40 drops		Sandalwood	35 drops
Grapefruit	25 drops		Oregano	30 drops
Pure Water	4 ounces		Pure Water	4 ounces

• • • • • •   • • • • • •

Lavender	40 drops		Copaiba	50 drops
Cedarwood (Atlas)	30 drops		Lavender	35 drops
Cardamom	30 drops		Spruce	25 drops
Fir Needles	30 drops		Thyme	20 drops
Fennel (Sweet)	20 drops		Frankincense	20 drops
Pure Water	4 ounces		Pure Water	4 ounces

STRESS REDUCERS

BATHS

Fill the bathtub with water as warm as you like. Mix the carrier oil with the essential oils and add to the bathwater. Disperse the oil evenly throughout the water. Enter the bath immediately, since the essential oils evaporate quickly. Breathe in the vapors deeply, relax, and enjoy your bath for 30 minutes.

Cedarwood (Atlas)	5 drops		Copaiba	7 drops
Lemon	5 drops		Elemi	5 drops
Palmarosa	5 drops		Orange	3 drops
Carrier Oil	1 teaspoon		Carrier Oil	1 teaspoon

Allspice	5 drops
Vanilla	5 drops
Chamomile (Roman)	5 drops
Carrier Oil	1 teaspoon

• • • • • • •

Lemon	5 drops
Lavender	5 drops
Patchouli	3 drops
Elemi	2 drops
Carrier Oil	1 teaspoon

• • • • • • •

Marjoram	4 drops
Bois de Rose	4 drops
Ylang-Ylang	4 drops
Cedarwood (Atlas)	3 drops
Carrier Oil	1 teaspoon

• • • • • • •

Geranium	5 drops
Cumin	4 drops
Petitgrain	4 drops
Ylang-Ylang	2 drops
Carrier Oil	1 teaspoon

Vanilla	5 drops
Fennel (Sweet)	4 drops
Lavender	4 drops
Nutmeg	2 drops
Carrier Oil	1 teaspoon

• • • • • • •

Sandalwood	5 drops
Spruce	5 drops
Frankincense	5 drops
Carrier Oil	1 teaspoon

• • • • • • •

Bois de Rose	4 drops
Cypress	4 drops
Tangerine	4 drops
Sandalwood	3 drops
Carrier Oil	1 teaspoon

• • • • • • •

Bergamot	5 drops
Allspice	4 drops
Copaiba	4 drops
Nutmeg	2 drops
Carrier Oil	1 teaspoon

DIFFUSOR

Depending on the type of diffusor you have, place the essential oils on the diffusor pad or in the glass bottle to disperse the aroma into the air.

Tangerine	50%		Lemon	50%
Lavender	40%		Juniper Berry	25%
Clary Sage	10%		Allspice	25%

Bergamot	40%		Petitgrain	30%
Cypress	40%		Chamomile (Roman)	30%
Palmarosa	20%		Lemongrass	20%
			Geranium	20%

• • • • • •

Cypress	30%		Petitgrain	40%
Spruce	30%		Allspice	20%
Mandarin	30%		Citronella	20%
Hyssop Decumbens	10%		Orange	20%

• • • • • •

Chamomile (Roman)	30%		Petitgrain	40%
Cypress	30%		Grapefruit	20%
Allspice	20%		Orange	20%
Clary Sage	10%		Hyssop Decumbens	20%
Geranium	10%			

MASSAGE

Massage into the abdomen, upper chest, back of the neck, and down the back until the oil is fully absorbed into the skin. Breathe in the vapors deeply. For best results, massage in the formula for 30 minutes.

Lavender	5 drops		Vetiver	5 drops
Cypress	4 drops		Marjoram	4 drops
Elemi	4 drops		Bergamot	4 drops
Lemongrass	4 drops		Nutmeg	4 drops
Juniper Berry	3 drops		Geranium	3 drops
Carrier Oil	4 teaspoons		Carrier Oil	4 teaspoons

• • • • • •

Mandarin	5 drops		Sandalwood	5 drops
Benzoin	4 drops		Myrtle	4 drops
Vanilla	4 drops		Cajeput	4 drops
Cedarwood (Atlas)	4 drops		Allspice	4 drops
Basil (Sweet)	3 drops		Oregano	3 drops
Carrier Oil	4 teaspoons		Carrier Oil	4 teaspoons

Tangerine	4 drops		Benzoin	5 drops
Labdanum	4 drops		Bois de Rose	4 drops
Lavender	4 drops		Clary Sage	4 drops
Copaiba	4 drops		Nutmeg	4 drops
Petitgrain	4 drops		Lemongrass	3 drops
Carrier Oil	4 teaspoons		Carrier Oil	4 teaspoons

• • • • • •   • • • • • •

Tangerine	5 drops		Peru Balsam	5 drops
Vetiver	4 drops		Citronella	4 drops
Grapefruit	4 drops		Copaiba	4 drops
Petitgrain	4 drops		Allspice	4 drops
Cajeput	3 drops		Juniper Berry	3 drops
Carrier Oil	4 teaspoons		Carrier Oil	4 teaspoons

• • • • • •   • • • • • •

Mandarin	5 drops		Peru Balsam	6 drops
Chamomile (Roman)	5 drops		Vanilla	5 drops
Spikenard	5 drops		Spikenard	5 drops
Lemon	5 drops		Cumin	4 drops
Carrier Oil	4 teaspoons		Carrier Oil	4 teaspoons

MIST SPRAYS

Fill a fine-mist spray bottle with purified water, then add the essential oils. Tighten the cap and shake well. Mist numerous times and breathe in the vapors deeply.

Orange	70 drops		Litsea Cubeba	40 drops
Cypress	50 drops		Copaiba	40 drops
Vetiver	30 drops		Petitgrain	35 drops
Pure Water	4 ounces		Vanilla	25 drops
			Pure Water	4 ounces

• • • • • •   • • • • • •

Orange	60 drops		Litsea Cubeba	50 drops
Dill	35 drops		Elemi	40 drops
Cedarwood (Atlas)	30 drops		Nutmeg	35 drops
Cypress	25 drops		Cumin	25 drops
Pure Water	4 ounces		Pure Water	4 ounces

Tangerine	60 drops		Lemongrass	40 drops
Myrtle	35 drops		Sandalwood	30 drops
Allspice	30 drops		Vanilla	30 drops
Cedarwood (Atlas)	25 drops		Allspice	30 drops
Copaiba	20 drops		Lavender	20 drops
Pure Water	4 ounces		Pure Water	4 ounces

• • • • • • •

Sandalwood	50 drops		Mandarin	60 drops
Bergamot	50 drops		Lemongrass	50 drops
Anise	25 drops		Allspice	35 drops
Allspice	25 drops		Patchouli	30 drops
Geranium	25 drops		Pure Water	4 ounces
Pure Water	4 ounces			

• • • • • • •

Peru Balsam	50 drops		Bergamot	40 drops
Petitgrain	50 drops		Lemongrass	30 drops
Chamomile (Roman)	50 drops		Grapefruit	30 drops
Pure Water	4 ounces		Patchouli	25 drops
			Cumin	25 drops
			Pure Water	4 ounces

SAUNA/STEAM ROOM—MIST SPRAYS

During stressful time periods, relax in a steam bath or sauna for 10 minute, breathing the vapors deeply, while misting the oils. Be sure to close your eyes when misting to avoid getting vapors in the eyes.

Lavender	50 drops		Lavender	70 drops
Copaiba	40 drops		Mandarin	30 drops
Litsea Cubeba	30 drops		Allspice	20 drops
Pure Water	4 ounces		Pure Water	4 ounces

• • • • • •

Cedarwood (Atlas)	60 drops		Fir Needles	30 drops
Tea Tree	30 drops		Coriander	30 drops
Orange	30 drops		Sandalwood	30 drops
Pure Water	4 ounces		Bois de Rose	30 drops
			Pure Water	4 ounces

Peppermint	50 drops	Cypress	50 drops
Juniper Berry	35 drops	Mandarin	40 drops
Copaiba	35 drops	Cajeput	30 drops
Pure Water	4 ounces	Pure Water	4 ounces

• • • • • • •

Sandalwood	40 drops	Spruce	50 drops
Eucalyptus	30 drops	Copaiba	30 drops
Pine	30 drops	Bay	20 drops
Thyme	20 drops	Ginger	20 drops
Pure Water	4 ounces	Pure Water	4 ounces

• • • • • • •

Sandalwood	40 drops	Ylang-Ylang	35 drops
Myrtle	40 drops	Cedarwood (Atlas)	35 drops
Spruce	40 drops	Cinnamon	30 drops
Pure Water	4 ounces	Ginger	20 drops
		Pure Water	4 ounces

• • • • • • (left)   • • • • • • (right)

Fir Needles	30 drops	Sandalwood	50 drops
Cypress	30 drops	Frankincense	30 drops
Cedarwood (Atlas)	30 drops	Cedarwood (Atlas)	20 drops
Chamomile (Roman)	30 drops	Orange	20 drops
Pure Water	4 ounces	Pure Water	4 ounces

YOGA

Yoga exercises have become popular in the West in recent years. The deep-breathing and stretching exercises are an excellent way to reduce stress.

APPLICATION

Apply one of these formulas on the muscles and joints you want to stretch, prior to doing the exercise.

Cedarwood (Atlas)	8 drops	Peru Balsam	10 drops
Lemon	7 drops	Palmarosa	5 drops
Ginger	5 drops	Eucalyptus	5 drops
Sesame	4 teaspoons	Sesame	4 teaspoons

Lemon	8 drops		Benzoin	8 drops
Copaiba	6 drops		Marjoram	6 drops
Oregano	6 drops		Spearmint	6 drops
Sesame	4 teaspoons		Sesame	4 teaspoons

• • • • • •   • • • • • •

Spearmint	8 drops		Tangerine	10 drops
Ginger	7 drops		Frankincense	5 drops
Juniper Berry	5 drops		Pepper (Black)	5 drops
Sesame	4 teaspoons		Sesame	4 teaspoons

• • • • • •   • • • • • •

Labdanum	10 drops		Vetiver	8 drops
Lime	5 drops		Pepper (Black)	7 drops
Ginger	5 drops		Ylang-Ylang	5 drops
Sesame	4 teaspoons		Sesame	4 teaspoons

• • • • • •   • • • • • •

Orange	6 drops		Cedarwood (Atlas)	8 drops
Copaiba	6 drops		Cardamom	6 drops
Peru Balsam	4 drops		Bois de Rose	6 drops
Vetiver	4 drops		Sesame	4 teaspoons
Sesame	4 teaspoons			

AROMA LAMPS

While doing yoga exercises, you will find the vapors from these formulas relaxing.

Fill the container with water, add the essential oils, then heat. Breathe in the vapors deeply.

Sandalwood	9 drops		Cedarwood (Atlas)	10 drops
Clove	6 drops		Spruce	10 drops
Cypress	5 drops			

• • • • • •   • • • • • •

Marjoram	10 drops		Lemon	7 drops
Orange	7 drops		Guaiacwood	7 drops
Spearmint	3 drops		Myrtle	3 drops
			Cedarwood (Atlas)	3 drops

Bois de Rose	10 drops		Cypress	8 drops
Lavender	5 drops		Sandalwood	7 drops
Spruce	5 drops		Clove	5 drops

• • • • • • •

Bois de Rose	7 drops		Bay	10 drops
Bay	7 drops		Myrtle	5 drops
Cedarwood (Atlas)	6 drops		Palmarosa	5 drops

• • • • • • •

Benzoin	7 drops		Guaiacwood	7 drops
Clove	7 drops		Spruce	7 drops
Lemongrass	6 drops		Lemongrass	6 drops

DIFFUSOR

Depending on the type of diffusor you have, place the essential oils on the diffusor pad or in the glass bottle to disperse the aroma into the air.

Frankincense	50%		Frankincense	30%
Orange	50%		Myrtle	30%
			Spruce	30%
			Anise	10%

• • • • • • (right column)

Lavender	50%		Marjoram	40%
Bois de Rose	50%		Orange	40%
			Juniper Berry	20%

Tangerine	50%		Petitgrain	40%
Bois de Rose	30%		Orange	35%
Juniper Berry	20%		Allspice	25%

Copaiba	50%		Spruce	40%
Orange	30%		Lemon	40%
Marjoram	10%		Cajeput	20%
Clove	10%			

Mandarin	50%	Tangerine	50%
Marjoram	30%	Bay	30%
Spearmint	20%	Grapefruit	20%

MIST SPRAYS

Select one of the formulas, and spray throughout the room before doing yoga exercises.

Fill the fine-mist spray bottle with purified water, then add the essential oils. Tighten the cap and shake well. Spray the mist many times in the room, prior to doing the exercises. Breathe in the vapors deeply.

Sandalwood	50 drops	Orange	40 drops
Orange	50 drops	Sandalwood	40 drops
Spruce	50 drops	Clove	40 drops
Pure Water	4 ounces	Cumin	30 drops
		Pure Water	4 ounces

• • • • • •

Cedarwood (Atlas)	75 drops	Cedarwood (Atlas)	70 drops
Lemongrass	65 drops	Spruce	50 drops
Sage	10 drops	Fir Needles	30 drops
Pure Water	4 ounces	Pure Water	4 ounces

• • • • • •

Copaiba	50 drops	Benzoin	70 drops
Cypress	30 drops	Thyme	30 drops
Bergamot	30 drops	Bergamot	30 drops
Citronella	30 drops	Spearmint	20 drops
Frankincense	10 drops	Pure Water	4 ounces
Pure Water	4 ounces		

• • • • • •

Sandalwood	50 drops	Bois de Rose	50 drops
Cinnamon Leaf	40 drops	Guaiacwood	35 drops
Allspice	20 drops	Anise	20 drops
Lemongrass	20 drops	Allspice	20 drops
Sage	10 drops	Sage	15 drops
Cumin	10 drops	Lavender	10 drops
Pure Water	4 ounces	Pure Water	4 ounces

Lavender	60 drops		Cinnamon Leaf	50 drops
Allspice	40 drops		Cedarwood (Atlas)	50 drops
Spearmint	20 drops		Tangerine	50 drops
Lemon	15 drops		Pure Water	4 ounces
Sandalwood	15 drops			
Pure Water	4 ounces			

CHAPTER 8

SHAPING UP

✪ ✪ ✪

LARGE NUMBERS OF people in the Western world are overweight. Many overweight people have cellulite deposits. These deposits are stored in the thighs, hips, buttocks, and arms, and appear as lumpy orange-peel-like skin. Cellulite buildup is not only undesirable from an aesthetic sense, but overweight people have a shorter life expectancy and are subject to numerous diseases and accidents. Overweight women have a greater number of fertility difficulties and suffer social and emotional problems as a result of their condition.

Many people go on weight-loss diets, but fail to achieve permanent results. Changing a habit that has been deeply ingrained over the years requires a strong commitment and unyielding determination. Emphasis should be placed on a longer-term approach with the focus on the main reason for eating—to nourish and maintain a healthy body.

EXERCISE

- Warm muscles by doing an aerobic exercise like walking before stretching, to help avoid the possibility of pulling a muscle or tearing ligaments.
- Breathing right makes exercising more enjoyable. Exhale on the exertion and inhale when relaxing. This synchronizes your natural breathing pattern with the motion of the exercise, requiring less effort.
- It is inaccurate to say that muscle turns to fat when inactive and fat turns into muscle with regular exercise. Exercise builds muscle and burns fat. If you let long periods of time lapse in between workouts, your muscles will shrink and fat may form on top of the muscles, making you look flabby.
- Workouts can be split up into 10-minute intervals throughout the day, instead of one of 30 minutes' duration.

Getting into shape is an achievement we can attain by keeping a good mental attitude, practicing visualization exercises, maintaining a proper diet, exercising, using mood-uplifting essential oils, and cellulite treatments.

FORMULAS

CELLULITE REDUCTION

Many people have cellulite. By eating a balanced diet of wholesome foods and using these cellulite-reducing blends, losing weight and inches is feasible.

BATHS

Fill the bathtub with water as warm as you like. Mix the essential oils with the carrier oil, pour the formula into the bathwater, and disperse throughout. Enter the bath immediately since the essential oils evaporate quickly. Enjoy your bath for 30 minutes.

Citronella	5 drops		Amyris	5 drops
Sandalwood	5 drops		Orange	5 drops
Grapefruit	5 drops		Lavender	5 drops
Carrier Oil	1 teaspoon		Carrier Oil	1 teaspoon

• • • • • •

Copaiba	5 drops		Bay	5 drops
Orange	5 drops		Lavender	5 drops
Ginger	3 drops		Patchouli	5 drops
Rosemary	2 drops		Carrier Oil	1 teaspoon
Carrier Oil	1 teaspoon			

• • • • • •

Litsea Cubeba	5 drops		Grapefruit	5 drops
Guaiacwood	5 drops		Copaiba	4 drops
Ginger	5 drops		Fennel (Sweet)	4 drops
Carrier oil	1 teaspoon		Juniper Berry	2 drops
			Carrier Oil	1 teaspoon

• • • • • •

Cypress	5 drops		Geranium	5 drops
Lemon	5 drops		Lemon	4 drops
Fennel (Sweet)	5 drops		Guaiacwood	4 drops
Carrier Oil	1 teaspoon		Rosemary	2 drops
			Carrier Oil	1 teaspoon

MASSAGE

Massage one of the formulas deeply into the cellulite area for at least 30 minutes. An hour after the massage, mix bentonite clay with apple cider vinegar into a liquidy paste. Use only glass or wooden utensils, since the clay is very absorbent and attracts toxic materials. Apply the paste on the cellulite area, and wait an hour for it to dry. Then take a bath and, without using soap, wash off the clay.

Litsea Cubeba	8 drops		Cypress	8 drops
Lemon	7 drops		Lime	5 drops
Celery	3 drops		Cedarwood (Atlas)	4 drops
Peru Balsam	2 drops		Pepper (Black)	3 drops
Carrier Oil	4 teaspoons		Carrier Oil	4 teaspoons

• • • • • •

Bay	4 drops		Copaiba	6 drops
Thyme	4 drops		Fennel (Sweet)	4 drops
Celery	4 drops		Juniper Berry	4 drops
Cedarwood (Atlas)	4 drops		Cinnamon Leaf	3 drops
Litsea Cubeba	4 drops		Tangerine	3 drops
Carrier Oil	4 teaspoons		Carrier Oil	4 teaspoons

• • • • • •

Litsea Cubeba	7 drops		Grapefruit	5 drops
Copaiba	7 drops		Fennel (Sweet)	5 drops
Pepper (Black)	6 drops		Patchouli	5 drops
Carrier Oil	4 teaspoons		Lime	5 drops
			Carrier Oil	4 teaspoons

• • • • • •

Benzoin	8 drops		Tangerine	7 drops
Celery	5 drops		Lemon	6 drops
Basil (Sweet)	4 drops		Patchouli	4 drops
Rosemary	3 drops		Juniper Berry	3 drops
Carrier Oil	4 teaspoons		Carrier Oil	4 teaspoons

Amyris	5 drops	Oregano	5 drops
Cedarwood (Atlas)	5 drops	Myrtle	5 drops
Geranium	5 drops	Celery	5 drops
Basil (Sweet)	5 drops	Amyris	5 drops
Carrier Oil	4 teaspoons	Carrier Oil	4 teaspoons

PRE-EXERCISE APPLICATION

Apply one of these formulas on your muscles one hour prior to doing your exercises. These formulas will help bring in circulation and loosen the muscles.

Ginger	5 drops	Ginger	6 drops
Peppermint	5 drops	Labdanum	6 drops
Copaiba	5 drops	Thyme	4 drops
Peru Balsam	5 drops	Pepper (Black)	4 drops
Sesame	4 teaspoons	Sesame	4 teaspoons

• • • • • • •

Peru Balsam	6 drops	Nutmeg	5 drops
Grapefruit	5 drops	Geranium	5 drops
Peppermint	5 drops	Copaiba	5 drops
Oregano	4 drops	Oregano	5 drops
Sesame	4 teaspoons	Sesame	4 teaspoons

• • • • • • •

Peru Balsam	6 drops	Benzoin	5 drops
Spearmint	5 drops	Bois de Rose	4 drops
Eucalyptus	4 drops	Oregano	4 drops
Ginger	3 drops	Grapefruit	4 drops
Lemon	2 drops	Spearmint	3 drops
Sesame	4 teaspoons	Sesame	4 teaspoons

• • • • • • •

Sandalwood	5 drops	Grapefruit	6 drops
Pepper (Black)	5 drops	Copaiba	6 drops
Copaiba	5 drops	Bois de Rose	6 drops
Peppermint	5 drops	Sandalwood	2 drops
Sesame	4 teaspoons	Sesame	4 teaspoons

BREATHE EASIER WHILE EXERCISING

These formulas will help you breathe more easily as you exercise.

APPLICATION

Apply one of these formulas to the upper chest, abdomen, and the back of the neck until the oil is absorbed into the skin. Breathe in the vapors deeply.

Copaiba	5 drops	Eucalyptus	4 drops
Spearmint	5 drops	Litsea Cubeba	3 drops
Carrier Oil	2 teaspoons	Cajeput	3 drops
		Carrier Oil	2 teaspoons

. . . .

Lime	5 drops	Frankincense	4 drops
Peppermint	3 drops	Eucalyptus	4 drops
Sandalwood	2 drops	Clove	2 drops
Carrier Oil	2 teaspoons	Carrier Oil	2 teaspoons

. . . .

Peppermint	5 drops	Lavender	4 drops
Cedarwood (Atlas)	3 drops	Spearmint	4 drops
Lavender	2 drops	Copaiba	2 drops
Carrier Oil	2 teaspoons	Carrier Oil	2 teaspoons

. . . .

Juniper Berry	3 drops	Oregano	3 drops
Copaiba	3 drops	Lime	3 drops
Hyssop Decumbens	2 drops	Spearmint	3 drops
Thyme	2 drops	Rosemary	1 drop
Carrier Oil	2 teaspoons	Carrier Oil	2 teaspoons

. . . .

Hyssop Decumbens	4 drops	Fir Needles	3 drops
Helichrysum	4 drops	Myrtle	3 drops
Cedarwood (Atlas)	2 drops	Cajeput	2 drops
Carrier Oil	2 teaspoons	Sandalwood	2 drops
		Carrier Oil	2 teaspoons

DIFFUSOR

Depending on the type of diffusor you have, place the essential oils on the diffusor pad or in the glass bottle to disperse the aroma into the air.

Lavender	50%		Clove	25%
Peppermint	50%		Myrtle	25%
			Cajeput	25%
			Bois de Rose	25%

· · · · · · ·

Pine	30%		Fir Needles	35%
Juniper Berry	30%		Eucalyptus	35%
Spruce	30%		Cypress	30%
Peppermint	10%			

· · · · · · ·

Spearmint	60%		Lavender	40%
Cajeput	40%		Clove	30%
			Juniper Berry	30%

MIST SPRAYS

Fill a fine-mist spray bottle with purified water, then add the essential oils. Tighten the cap and shake well. Mist numerous times and breathe in the vapors deeply.

Cedarwood (Atlas)	40 drops		Copaiba	40 drops
Citronella	40 drops		Eucalyptus	40 drops
Clove	40 drops		Spearmint	40 drops
Thyme	30 drops		Lemon	30 drops
Pure Water	4 ounces		Pure Water	4 ounces

· · · · · ·

Tea Tree	50 drops		Myrtle	40 drops
Lime	50 drops		Peppermint	40 drops
Sandalwood	50 drops		Copaiba	40 drops
Pure Water	4 ounces		Grapefruit	30 drops
			Pure Water	4 ounces

Lavender	50 drops		Fir Needles	50 drops
Cypress	50 drops		Litsea Cubeba	50 drops
Eucalyptus	50 drops		Spruce	50 drops
Pure Water	4 ounces		Pure Water	4 ounces

FOOD AND DIET

Many people in the world do not have an adequate choice of foods available to eat. They may live in countries where supplies are limited or they may not be able to afford foods that provide proper nutrition for good health. In Western countries, people are fortunate to have an enormous availability and variety of foods to select from.

SUGGESTED FOOD GROUPS

Grains: Whole grains are the staff of life and provide an important part of our nutritional needs. Every culture includes at least one grain that forms the mainstay of the diet. Whole grains are vital to daily nutrition. At least 60 percent of the diet should consist of whole, unrefined grains.

Legumes: Lentils and beans supply the body with essential protein and complex carbohydrates. Fifteen percent of the diet should consist of legumes.

Seaweed: Seaweed is a rich source of nutrients and has been a staple food in the Orient for centuries. Sea vegetables should be included in the daily diet.

Oils: It is recommended to use minimum heat when sautéing. Use only small amounts to flavor foods. The maximum is one teaspoon per day.

Fruits and Vegetables: Fresh, organically grown produce provides the body with many vital nutrients and enzymes. It is best to eat these foods when they are in season. Fifteen to 20 percent of the diet should consist of vegetables; fruits should be eaten sparingly. Unsulfured dried fruits are permissible.

Water: Avoid constant drinking throughout the day; drink when thirsty. Purified or well water is recommended.

The food selection and meals are in accordance with the macrobiotic approach to attaining a healthy body. The philosophy and principles of macrobiotic living were initially developed by George Ohsawa. Michio Kushi studied under George Ohsawa, and is responsible for the further expansion and advancement of the teachings.

RECOMMENDED FOODS

WHOLE GRAINS
amaranth
barley
brown rice
buckwheat
kamut
millet
oats
quinoa
rye
spelt
teff
whole wheat

LEGUMES
adzuki beans
black beans
black-eyed peas
black soy beans
garbanzo beans
kidney beans
lentils
mung beans
navy beans
pinto beans
split peas

SEAWEED
agar
arame
bladderwrack
dulse
hijiki
Irish moss
kelp
kombu
nori
wakame

VEGETABLES
bok choy
broccoli
burdock root
cabbage
carrots
cauliflower
celery
daikon radish
dandelion
endive
escarole
garlic
ginger
Jerusalem artichokes
kale
kohlrabi
leeks
onions
parsnips
pumpkin
radishes
romaine lettuce
shiitake mushrooms
string beans
turnips
watercress
winter squash

SOY PRODUCTS
miso
soy sauce**
tamari sauce**
tofu

OILS
flaxseed
sesame
safflower
sunflower

SEEDS*
pumpkin
sesame
sunflower

FRUITS*
apples
apricots
berries
cantaloupe
grapes
honeydew melon
peaches
pears
persimmons
plums
strawberries
watermelon

FISH
carp
cod
flounder
haddock
smelt
snapper
sole
trout

NUTS
almonds
chestnuts
filberts
pecans
pine nuts
walnuts

* Use sparingly.
** Choose the product without alcohol as an ingredient and use sparingly.

Sample Menus

* All foods should be cooked on a low flame for several hours until done.
* Use stainless steel, glass cookware, or a Crock pot.
* Eat as much as you wish, without overeating.

BREAKFAST

CHOICE #1

Choose from one or a combination of these grains:

Millet, buckwheat, whole wheat, oats, quinoa, or *spelt*

Purified water

Unrefined sea salt

Choose from these fruits, dry or fresh:

Raisins, peaches, apricots, apples, pears, persimmons, or *berries*

Preparation: Cook the whole grain cereal in water with a pinch of sea salt together with the dried fruit, or add fresh fruit after cooking.

CHOICE #2

Choose from one or a combination of these grains:

Millet, buckwheat, whole wheat, oats, quinoa, or *spelt*

Purified water

Unrefined sea salt (optional)

Chopped almonds

Flaxseeds

Essential oil of cinnamon

Preparation: Cook the whole grain cereal in water with a pinch of sea salt. Then add chopped almonds, flaxseeds, and stir in well one drop of the essential oil of cinnamon into the cereal.

LUNCH

CHOICE #1

Fish
Ginger (chopped into small pieces)
Toasted sesame seeds (Powder the seeds in a grinder, add sea salt, to taste, a drop of the
    essential oil of basil [sweet], and mix well. Bake for 25 minutes at 250°F [120°C],
    until lightly toasted.)
Soy sauce
Brown rice
Purified water
Unrefined sea salt (optional)
Essential oil of oregano
Daikon radish
Carrots

Preparation: Place the fish in a baking pan, put it in the oven to broil, and set the temperature at 300°F (150°C). When the fish is almost done, add chopped ginger and toasted sesame seed powder on top and lightly pour soy sauce over it.

Cook brown rice in purified water with a pinch of sea salt. When done, add one drop of the essential oil of oregano and mix well. Steam the daikon radish with carrots until tender. Serve the rice and steamed vegetables with the fish.

CHOICE #2

Cabbage
Broccoli
Brown rice
Split peas
Purified water
Unrefined sea salt (optional)
Toasted sesame seeds (Powder the seeds in a grinder, add sea salt, to taste, a drop of the
    essential oil of oregano, and mix well. Bake for 25 minutes at 250°F [120°C], until
    lightly toasted.)

Preparation: Cook the cabbage, broccoli, brown rice, and split peas in purified water and add a pinch of sea salt. When done, mix a generous amount of toasted sesame seed powder into the food.

DINNER

CHOICE #1

Tofu (sliced thin)

Toasted sesame seeds (Powder the seeds in a grinder, add sea salt, to taste, a drop of the essential oil of oregano, and mix well. Bake for 25 minutes at 250°F [120°C], until lightly toasted.)

Sunflower seeds

Soy sauce

Onion (sliced)

Lettuce

Carrots (sliced into sticks)

Celery (sliced into sticks)

Preparation: Place the slices of tofu in a baking pan. Sprinkle some toasted sesame seed powder and sunflower seeds on top of the tofu, then lightly pour soy sauce over it. Place the pan in the oven, set the temperature at 250°F (120°C), and broil for about 20–30 minutes. Serve with a salad of lettuce, carrots, and celery sticks.

CHOICE #2

Kombu (seaweed)

Adzuki beans

Split peas

Mung beans

Purified water

Soy sauce

Toasted sesame seeds (Powder the seeds in a grinder with sea salt, to taste, a drop of the essential oil of cardamom, and mix well. Bake for 25 minutes on 250°F [120°C], until lightly toasted. As it cools, stir in 10 drops of flaxseed oil.)

Garlic (chopped into small pieces)

Lettuce

Carrots (sliced into sticks)

Celery (sliced into sticks)

Preparation: Cook the kombu (seaweed), adzuki beans, split peas, and mung beans in purified water on a low flame for four hours. Before removing from heat add soy sauce, to taste. As the food cools, add some toasted sesame seed powder, garlic pieces, and mix well. Serve with fresh salad of lettuce, carrots, and celery sticks.

CHAPTER 9

ESSENTIAL OIL PROFILES

❂ ❂ ❂

ALLSPICE (PIMENTO BERRY)

Botanical name: *Pimenta Officinalis*
Scent: Clove-like
Allspice is an evergreen tree that grows to 30–70 feet and has leathery leaves and small white flowers that develop into aromatic berries. The berries turn black when ripe.

EFFECTS ON THE MIND AND EMOTIONS

calming
mood uplifting
improves mental clarity and memory
promotes a restful sleep
reduces stress

EFFECTS ON THE BODY

warming
relaxes tight muscles
lessens pain
the vapors help breathing
improves digestion
helps in the reduction of cellulite deposits
purifying

OTHER USES

disinfectant
Precaution: Essential oil of allspice can irritate the skin.

AMYRIS

Botanical name: *Amyris Balsamifera*
Scent: Smokey sweet
Amyris is an evergreen tree growing to about 60 feet with clusters of white flowers that develop into edible bluish-black fruit.

EFFECTS ON THE MIND AND EMOTIONS

calming
promotes a peaceful state of mind
releases anxiety

EFFECTS ON THE BODY

cooling
purifying

OTHER USES

fixative for fragrances

ANISE

Botanical name: *Pimpinella Anisum*
Scent: Licorice-like
Anise reaches a height of about two feet and has small white flowers.

EFFECTS ON THE MIND AND EMOTIONS

calming
promotes restful sleep

EFFECTS ON THE BODY
lessens pain
the vapors help breathing
improves digestion
stimulates lactation in nursing mothers
Precaution: Essential oil of anise is stupefying
in large amounts.

BASIL (SWEET)

Botanical name: *Ocimum Basilicum*
Scent: Licorice
Basil is a bushy plant that grows to two feet
and has white, blue, or purple flowers.
About 150 varieties of basil exist.

EFFECTS ON THE MIND AND EMOTIONS
calming
mood uplifting
helps relieve mental fatigue in small amounts
improves mental clarity and memory
promotes restful sleep
sharpens the senses
reduces stress
helpful for meditation

EFFECTS ON THE BODY
cooling
lessens pain
improves digestion
stimulates lactation in nursing mothers
helpful in the reduction of cellulite deposits
purifying

OTHER USES
soothes the skin after insect bites

Precaution: Essential oil of basil can irritate
the skin. In large amounts the oil can be
toxic.

BAY (WEST INDIAN)

Botanical name: *Pimenta Racemosa* or
Pimenta Acris
Scent: Spicy
Bay is a tropical evergreen tree that grows to
about 30–50 feet. The tree has aromatic leathery leaves and clusters of white or pink flowers
that develop into black or purple oval berries.

EFFECTS ON THE MIND AND EMOTIONS
calming
improves mental clarity, alertness, and memory
sharpens the senses
promotes restful sleep
reduces stress

EFFECTS ON THE BODY
warming
relaxes tight muscles
soothing to sprains
lessens pain
the vapors help breathing
improves digestion
promotes perspiration
helps in the reduction of cellulite deposits
purifying

OTHER USES
disinfectant
repels insects
Precaution: Essential oil of bay can irritate
the skin.

BENZOIN

Botanical name: *Styrax Benzoin* or *Styrax Tonkinensis*

Scent: Cinnamon-vanilla

The benzoin tree grows to about 115 feet and has fragrant white flowers. The trunk secretes an aromatic resin when injured. The resin is also known as gum benjamin.

EFFECTS ON THE MIND AND EMOTIONS

calming
mood uplifting
promotes restful sleep
reduces stress
helpful for meditation

EFFECTS ON THE BODY

warming
relaxes tight muscles
breaks up congestion
reduces inflammation
improves the breathing
helps in the reduction of cellulite deposits
purifying
healing to the skin

OTHER USES

preservative in cosmetics
fixative for fragrances

BERGAMOT

Botanical name: *Citrus Bergamia*

Scent: Citrus

Bergamot is an evergreen citrus tree that grows to a height of about 15 feet and bears green to yellow fruit.

EFFECTS ON THE MIND AND EMOTIONS

calming
promotes restful sleep
mood uplifting
relieves anxiety, nervous tension, and stress
helps relieve mental fatigue
improves mental clarity and alertness
sharpens the senses
refreshing
balances the nervous system

EFFECTS ON THE BODY

cooling
helps in the reduction of cellulite deposits
purifying

OTHER USES

disinfectant

Precaution: Essential oil of bergamot can irritate dry skin. Skin can burn if exposed to sunlight after topical application.

BOIS DE ROSE (ROSEWOOD)

Botanical name: *Aniba Rosaeodora*

Scent: Slightly rosy

Bois de Rose is a large evergreen tree with yellow flowers.

EFFECTS ON THE MIND AND EMOTIONS

calming
mood uplifting
relieves nervousness and stress

EFFECTS ON THE BODY

lessens pain
regenerates and moisturizes the skin

CAJEPUT

Botanical name: *Melaleuca Leucadendron* or *Melalleuca Cajuputi*
Scent: Camphor-like
Cajeput is an evergreen tree that grows to a height of 50–100 feet. The tree is cultivated in many areas as an ornamental for its outstanding white, pink, or purple flowers. It belongs to a family of over 150 trees.

EFFECTS ON THE MIND AND EMOTIONS
calming
promotes restful sleep
reduces stress

EFFECTS ON THE BODY
slightly warming
relieves muscle aches and pains
breaks up congestion
the vapors help breathing

OTHER USES
disinfectant
repels insects

CARDAMOM

Botanical name: *Elettaria Cardamomum*
Scent: Spicy
Cardamom grows to a height of about 10 feet and has small yellow flowers that develop into a fruit with seeds inside.

EFFECTS ON THE MIND AND EMOTIONS
mood uplifting
improves mental clarity and memory
energizing

EFFECTS ON THE BODY
warming
relieves pain
improves physical strength
improves digestion

CEDARWOOD (ATLAS)

Botanical name: *Cedrus Atlantica*
Scent: Woody
Cedarwood is an evergreen tree that grows to a height of about 130 feet and has needle-like leaves. These trees can reach an age of 1000–2000 years if undisturbed.

EFFECTS ON THE MIND AND EMOTIONS
calming
promotes restful sleep
relieves anxiety and tension
helpful for meditation

EFFECTS ON THE BODY
cooling
relaxes tight muscles
lessens pain
the vapors help breathing
helps in the reduction of cellulite deposits
purifying

OTHER USES
repels insects

CELERY

Botanical name: *Apium Graveolens*
Scent: Strong celery
Celery grows to a height of one to two feet and has white flowers.

EFFECTS ON THE MIND AND EMOTIONS
cooling
calming
promotes restful sleep

EFFECTS ON THE BODY
helps in the reduction of cellulite deposits
purifying
Precaution: Essential oil of celery is very cleansing to the tissues; best used in small amounts due to its detoxifying properties.

CHAMOMILE (ROMAN)

Botanical name: *Anthemis Nobilis*
Scent: Apple-like
Chamomile grows to a height of about one foot and has small, daisy-like flowerheads.

EFFECTS ON THE MIND AND EMOTIONS
calming
mood uplifting
promotes restful sleep
reduces stress and tension

EFFECTS ON THE BODY
lessens pain
reduces inflammation
improves digestion
healing to the skin

OTHER USES
soothes the skin after insect bites

CINNAMON LEAF

Botanical name: *Cinnamomum Zeylanicum*
Scent: Cinnamon

The cinnamon tree grows to a height of about 50 feet and has leathery leaves and small white flowers that develop into light-blue berries.

EFFECTS ON THE MIND AND EMOTIONS
mood uplifting
helps relieve mental fatigue
reduces stress
reviving

EFFECTS ON THE BODY
warming
relaxes tight muscles
lessens pain
improves digestion
helps in the reduction of cellulite deposits
purifying

OTHER USES
disinfectant
repels insects
Precaution: Essential oil of cinnamon can irritate the skin.

CITRONELLA

Botanical name: *Cymbopogan Nardus*
Scent: Lemony
Citronella is an aromatic tall grass.

EFFECTS ON THE MIND AND EMOTIONS
calming
mood uplifting
improves mental clarity and alertness
reduces stress
mental stimulant

EFFECTS ON THE BODY
cooling

OTHER USES
repels insects

CLARY SAGE

Botanical name: *Salvia Sclarea*
Scent: Sweet and spicy
Clary sage grows to a height of about three feet. The flowers are pink, white, or blue, depending on the variety.

EFFECTS ON THE MIND AND EMOTIONS
calming
mood uplifting
promotes restful sleep
relieves stress and tension
aphrodisiac
encourages communication

EFFECTS ON THE BODY
lessens pain
improves digestion
contains a hormone-like substance similar to estrogen
Precaution: Essential oil of clary sage can be stupefying in large amounts.

CLOVE

Botanical name: *Eugenia Caryophyllata*
Scent: Hot and spicy
Clove is an evergreen tree that grows to about 40 feet and has bright pink buds that develop into yellow flowers, then into purple berries.

EFFECTS ON THE MIND AND EMOTIONS
mood uplifting
helps relieve mental fatigue
improves mental clarity and memory
reviving
aphrodisiac

EFFECTS ON THE BODY
warming
relieves pain
the vapors help breathing
improves digestion

OTHER USES
disinfectant
repels insects
Precaution: Essential oil of clove can irritate the skin.

COPAIBA

Botanical name: *Copaifera Officinalis*
Scent: Woody
The copaiba tree grows to about 50 feet.

EFFECTS ON THE MIND AND EMOTIONS
calming
promotes a peaceful state of mind
mood uplifting
improves mental clarity and alertness
promotes restful sleep
reduces stress and tension
helpful for meditation

EFFECTS ON THE BODY
warming
opens breathing passages
soothing to the intestines

allows deeper breathing
healing to the skin

Other Uses
fixative for fragrances

CORIANDER

Botanical name: *Coriandrum Sativum*
Scent: Musky
Coriander grows to a height of about three
feet and has small white flowers that develop
into green seeds. Coriander is also known as
cilantro, or Chinese parsley.

Effects on the Mind and Emotions
helps relieve mental fatigue
improves mental clarity and memory
reviving
energizing

Effects on the Body
relieves pain
improves digestion

CUBEB

Botanical name: *Piper Cubeba*
Scent: Peppery
Cubeb is an evergreen climbing woody
shrub that grows to a height of about 20 feet
and has clusters of flowers that develop into
small berries resembling peppers.

Effects on the Body
relieves pain
breaks up congestion
reduces inflammation

the vapors help breathing
improves digestion

CUMIN

Botanical name: *Cuminum Cyminum*
Scent: Strong spicy
Cumin grows to a height of about one foot,
has thread-like leaves, small white or pink
flowers, and aromatic seeds.

Effects on the Mind and Emotions
calming
mood uplifting
helps relieve mental fatigue
reduces stress
reviving
helpful for meditation

Effects on the Body
warming
relieves pain
improves digestion
helps in the reduction of cellulite deposits
purifying

CYPRESS

Botanical name: *Cupressus Sempervirens*
Scent: Woody
Cypress is an evergreen tree that grows to a
height of about 160 feet. Some trees are
believed to be older than 3000 years.

Effects on the Mind and Emotions
calming
mood uplifting
improves mental clarity and alertness

promotes restful sleep
reduces stress and nervous tension
refreshing
balances the nervous system

EFFECTS ON THE BODY
relaxes the muscles
reduces perspiration
contains a hormone-like substance similar to
     estrogen
helps in the reduction of cellulite deposits
purifying
contracts weak connective tissue
tones the skin

DILL

Botanical name: *Anethum Graveolens*
Scent: Spicy
Dill grows to a height of about three feet
and has small yellow flowers.

EFFECTS ON THE MIND AND EMOTIONS
calming
promotes restful sleep

EFFECTS ON THE BODY
relieves pain
improves digestion

OTHER USES
repels insects

ELEMI

Botanical name: *Canarium Luzonicum*
Scent: Lemon-like balsamic
Elemi is an evergreen tree that grows to a

height of about 100 feet and has yellow fragrant flowers that develop into green fruits
with nuts inside called pili nuts. These nuts
are a valuable food for millions of people.

EFFECTS ON THE MIND AND EMOTIONS
calming
mood uplifting
promotes restful sleep
reduces stress
helps to communicate feelings
helpful for meditation

EFFECTS ON THE BODY
warming
opens the breathing passages
healing to the skin

EUCALYPTUS

Botanical name: *Eucalyptus Globulus*
Scent: Fresh camphor-like
The eucalyptus tree is one of the tallest trees,
reaching over 300 feet and as high as 480
feet. The leaves are fragrant and leathery, the
flowers are white, and the fruit is contained
in a capsule. There are approximately 700
different species of eucalyptus.

EFFECTS ON THE MIND AND EMOTIONS
helps relieve mental fatigue
improves mental clarity and alertness
refreshing
reviving
energizing
stimulating

EFFECTS ON THE BODY

cooling

relieves pain and aching sore muscles

breaks up congestion

reduces inflammation

the vapors help breathing

OTHER USES

disinfectant

repels insects

Precaution: Essential oil of eucalyptus can be toxic in large amounts.

FENNEL

Botanical name: *Foeniculum Vulgare*

Scent: Strong licorice

Fennel grows to a height of three to seven feet and has green feathery leaves and clusters of small yellow flowers.

EFFECTS ON THE MIND AND EMOTIONS

calming

promotes restful sleep

reduces stress

EFFECTS ON THE BODY

warming

relieves pain

improves digestion

contains a hormone-like substance similar to estrogen

stimulates lactation in nursing mothers

helps in the reduction of cellulite deposits

purifying

OTHER USES

disinfectant

repels insects

Precaution: Essential oil of fennel can be stupefying in large amounts.

FIR NEEDLES

Botanical name: *Abies Balsamea*

Scent: Pine-like

Fir needles is an evergreen tree that grows to a height of about 40–80 feet and has needle-like leaves. There are approximately 40 species of the tree.

EFFECTS ON THE MIND AND EMOTIONS

calming

mood uplifting

improves mental clarity

refreshing

reviving

encourages communication

EFFECTS ON THE BODY

lessens pain

the vapors help breathing

helps in the reduction of cellulite

purifying

FRANKINCENSE

Botanical name: *Boswellia Thurifera*

Scent: Woody and camphor-like

Frankincense is a small tree that grows to about 20 feet and has white flowers.

EFFECTS ON THE MIND AND EMOTIONS

calming

mood uplifting

promotes restful sleep

encourages communication

brings out feelings

helpful for meditation

EFFECTS ON THE BODY

reduces inflammation

healing to the skin (reduces wrinkles)

GERANIUM

Botanical name: *Pelargonium Graveolens*

Scent: Rose-like

Geranium grows to a height of about three feet. There are over 700 species of the plant.

EFFECTS ON THE MIND AND EMOTIONS

calming in small amounts

stimulating in large amounts

mood uplifting

reduces stress and tension

encourages communication

EFFECTS ON THE BODY

cooling

lessens pain

reduces inflammation

helps in the reduction of cellulite deposits

purifying

soothes itching skin

OTHER USES

disinfectant

soothes the skin after insect bites

repels insects

GINGER

Botanical name: *Zingiber Officinale*

Scent: Spicy

Ginger grows to a height of about three feet and has white or yellow flowers.

EFFECTS ON THE MIND AND EMOTIONS

mood uplifting

helps relieve mental fatigue

improves mental clarity and memory

stimulating

EFFECTS ON THE BODY

warming

relaxes tight muscles

relieves aches and pains

improves digestion

relieves travel dizziness and nausea

OTHER USES

disinfectant

GRAPEFRUIT

Botanical name: *Citrus Paradisi*

Scent: Citrus

Grapefruit is an evergreen citrus tree that grows to a height of about 30–50 feet and has fragrant white flowers that develop into an edible fruit.

EFFECTS ON THE MIND AND EMOTIONS

mood uplifting

helps relieve mental fatigue

improves mental clarity, alertness, and memory

sharpens the senses

reduces stress

refreshing
reviving
energizing

EFFECTS ON THE BODY
cooling
increases physical strength and energy
helps in the reduction of cellulite deposits
purifying
Precaution: Essential oil of grapefruit can
irritate dry skin. Skin can burn if exposed to
sunlight after topical application.

GUAIACWOOD

Botanical name: *Guaiacum Officinale*
Scent: Sweet dried fruit
Guaiacwood is an evergreen tree that grows
to a height of about 40 feet and has leathery
leaves and blue or purple flowers.

EFFECTS ON THE MIND AND EMOTIONS
calming
helpful for meditation

EFFECTS ON THE BODY
reduces inflammation
purifying
healing to the skin

HELICHRYSUM

Botanical name: *Helichrysum Italicum* or
Helichrysum Angustifolium
Scent: Strong sweet
Helichrysum is an evergreen plant that
grows to a height of about two feet and has
daisy-like yellow flowers.

EFFECTS ON THE MIND AND EMOTIONS
calming
mood uplifting
improves mental clarity and alertness
reduces stress
reviving
euphoric

EFFECTS ON THE BODY
cooling
helps the breathing
increases muscle endurance

OTHER USES
disinfectant

HYSSOP DECUMBENS

Botanical name: *Hyssopus Officinalis, var.
Decumbens*
Scent: Sweet camphorous
Hyssop decumbens is semi-evergreen plant
that grows to a height of about one to four
feet and has aromatic leaves and spikes of
white, pink, blue, or dark purple flowers.

EFFECTS ON THE MIND AND EMOTIONS
calming
mood uplifting
improves mental clarity and alertness
reviving

EFFECTS ON THE BODY
the vapors help breathing

JUNIPER BERRY

Botanical name: *Juniperus Communis*
Scent: Evergreen forest
Juniper is an evergreen bush two to six feet high that sometimes reaches 25 feet, with silvery-green needle-like leaves. The green berries take three years to ripen to a blue color. The maximum lifespan of the bush is 2000 years.

EFFECTS ON THE MIND AND EMOTIONS
relaxing
mood uplifting
improves mental clarity and memory
reduces stress
refreshing
reviving

EFFECTS ON THE BODY
lessens pain
reduces inflammation
cleanses the intestines
helps in the reduction of cellulite deposits
purifying

OTHER USES
disinfectant
soothes the skin after insect bites
repels insects
Precaution: Essential oil of juniper, if used in large amounts, can cause the body to become dehydrated.

LABDANUM (CISTUS)

Botanical name: *Cistus Ladaniferus*
Scent: Sweet prune-like
Labdanum is a small evergreen bush that grows to a height of about 10 feet and has large white flowers.

EFFECTS ON THE MIND AND EMOTIONS
calming
mood uplifting
promotes restful sleep
reduces stress
encourages communication
brings out feelings
helpful for meditation

EFFECTS ON THE BODY
warming
loosens tight muscles

OTHER USES
fixative for fragrances

LAVENDER

Botanical name: *Lavandula Officinalis* or *Lavandula Augustifolia*
Scent: Floral herbaceous
Lavender is an evergreen plant that grows to a height of about three feet and has lilac-colored flowers. There are 28 species of this plant.

EFFECTS ON THE MIND AND EMOTIONS
calming in small amounts
stimulating in large amounts
mood uplifting
promotes restful sleep
reduces stress and tension
soothing for the nervous system
balances mood swings

EFFECTS ON THE BODY

relaxes tight muscles
lessens aches and pains
breaks up congestion
reduces inflammation
the vapors help breathing
improves digestion
soothing to the intestines
helps in the reduction of cellulite
purifying
healing to the skin

OTHER USES

disinfectant
soothes the skin after insect bites
repels insects

LEMON

Botanical name: *Citrus Limonum*
Scent: Lemony
Lemon is an evergreen citrus tree that grows
to a height of 10–20 feet and has white, fragrant flowers that develop into edible fruits.

EFFECTS ON THE MIND AND EMOTIONS

calming
mood uplifting
helps relieve mental fatigue
improves mental clarity, alertness, and memory
sharpens the senses
promotes restful sleep
reduces stress
refreshing
reviving
balancing; calming or energizing
balances the nervous system

EFFECTS ON THE BODY

cooling
helps in the reduction of cellulite deposits
purifying

OTHER USES

disinfectant
soothes the skin after insect bites
Precaution: Essential oil of lemon can irritate
dry skin. Skin can burn if exposed to sunlight after topical application.

LEMONGRASS

Botanical name: *Cymbopogon Citratus*
Scent: Strong lemon
Lemongrass is a grass that grows to about
two feet and has bulbous stems and sword-
like leaves.

EFFECTS ON THE MIND AND EMOTIONS

mood uplifting
improves alertness
promotes restful sleep
reduces stress
refreshing
reviving
balances the nervous system

EFFECTS ON THE BODY

reduces inflammation
the vapors help breathing
improves digestion
stimulates lactation in nursing mothers
contracts weak connective tissue
tones the skin

OTHER USES
disinfectant
repels insects
Precaution: Essential oil of lemongrass can irritate dry skin.

LIME

Botanical name: *Citrus Limetta*
Scent: Fresh citrus
Lime is an evergreen citrus tree that grows to about 10 feet and has fragrant white flowers that develop into edible fruits.

EFFECTS ON THE MIND AND EMOTIONS
mood uplifting
helps relieve mental fatigue
improves mental clarity, alertness, and memory
sharpens the senses
reduces stress
refreshing
reviving
strengthening to the nerves

EFFECTS ON THE BODY
cooling
helps in the reduction of cellulite deposits
purifying

OTHER USES
disinfectant
soothes the skin after insect bites
Precaution: Essential oil of lime can irritate dry skin. Skin can burn if exposed to sunlight after topical application.

LITSEA CUBEBA

Botanical name: *Litsea Cubeba*
Scent: Lemony
Litsea cubeba is an evergreen tree that grows to about 30 feet and has white flowers that develop into small red or black berries.

EFFECTS ON THE MIND AND EMOTIONS
calming
mood uplifting
improves mental clarity, alertness, and memory
promotes restful sleep
refreshing
reviving
euphoric
encourages communication

EFFECTS ON THE BODY
cooling
relieves pain
improves digestion

MANDARIN

Botanical name: *Citrus Nobilis*
Scent: Sweet citrus
Mandarin is an evergreen tree that grows to a height of about 25 feet and has fragrant flowers that develop into edible fruits.

EFFECTS ON THE MIND AND EMOTIONS
calming
promotes restful sleep
mood uplifting
improves mental clarity and alertness
sharpens the senses
relieves stress and tension

EFFECTS ON THE BODY

cooling

helps in the reduction of cellulite deposits

purifying

Precaution: Essential oil of mandarin can irritate dry skin. Skin can burn if exposed to sunlight after topical application.

MARJORAM

Botanical name: *Origanum Majorana* or *Majorana Hortensis*

Scent: Spicy

Marjoram is a bushy plant that grows to a height of about two feet and has white or purple flowers and light-green leaves.

EFFECTS ON THE MIND AND EMOTIONS

calming

promotes restful sleep

EFFECTS ON THE BODY

warming

relaxes tight muscles

relieves aches and pains

breaks up congestion

reduces inflammation

the vapors help breathing

improves digestion

OTHER USES

disinfectant

soothes the skin after insect bites

MYRRH

Botanical name: *Commiphora Myrrha*

Scent: Balsamic

Myrrh is a small tree growing to about nine feet.

EFFECTS ON THE MIND AND EMOTIONS

calming

mood uplifting

promotes restful sleep

helpful for meditation

EFFECTS ON THE BODY

cooling

reduces inflammation

healing to the skin

OTHER USES

fixative for fragrances

MYRTLE

Botanical name: *Myrtus Communis*

Scent: Fresh camphor-like

Myrtle is an evergreen shrub that grows to a height of 10–18 feet and has scented leaves and small aromatic white blossoms. The flowers develop into bluish-black berries that are edible fresh or dried. There are about 16 species of the myrtle shrub.

EFFECTS ON THE MIND AND EMOTIONS

calming

mood uplifting

refreshing

helpful for meditation

EFFECTS ON THE BODY
relieves pain
the vapors help breathing

NEROLI

Botanical name: *Citrus Aurantium*
Scent: Sweet floral
Neroli is from the fragrant white blossoms
of the bitter-orange tree.

EFFECTS ON THE MIND AND EMOTIONS
calming
mood uplifting
reduces nervous tension

NUTMEG

Botanical name: *Myristica Fragrans*
Scent: Spicy
Nutmeg is an evergreen tree that grows to a
height of 60–80 feet and has large, fragrant
leaves and small yellow flowers that develop
into yellow fruits. The flowers of the female
tree bear fruit after being pollinated by the
flowers of the male tree.

EFFECTS ON THE MIND AND EMOTIONS
calming and promotes restful sleep in small
    amounts
stimulating in large amounts
mood uplifting
improves mental clarity and alertness
reviving

EFFECTS ON THE BODY
slightly warming
relaxes tight muscles

relieves aches and pains
improves digestion
Precaution: Essential oil of nutmeg can be
stupefying in large amounts.

ORANGE

Botanical name: *Citrus Aurantium* or *Citrus
Sinensis*
Scent: Sweet orange
Orange is an evergreen citrus tree that grows
to a height of about 25 feet and has fragrant
white flowers that develop into edible fruits.

EFFECTS ON THE MIND AND EMOTIONS
calming
mood uplifting
promotes restful sleep
improves mental clarity
reduces stress

EFFECTS ON THE BODY
cooling
helps in the reduction of cellulite deposits
purifying
Precaution: Essential oil of orange can irritate dry skin. Skin can burn if exposed to
sunlight after topical application.

OREGANO

Botanical name: *Origanum Vulgare*
Scent: Spicy
Oregano grows to a height of one to two
feet and has dark green leaves and purple
buds that blossom into white, pink, or lilac-
colored flowers. The entire plant is aromatic.
There are about 20 species of oregano.

EFFECTS ON THE MIND AND EMOTIONS
mood uplifting
improves mental clarity and alertness

EFFECTS ON THE BODY
warming
loosens tight muscles
relieves muscle aches and pains
increases physical endurance and energy
the vapors help breathing
improves digestion
promotes perspiration
helps in the reduction of cellulite deposits
purifying

OTHER USES
disinfectant
repels insects
Precaution: Essential oil of oregano can irritate the skin.

PALMAROSA

Botanical name: *Cymbopogon Martini*
Scent: Sweet
Palmarosa is a fragrant grass.

EFFECTS ON THE MIND AND EMOTIONS
calming
mood uplifting
reduces stress
refreshing

EFFECTS ON THE BODY
warming
lessens aches and pains
reduces inflammation
regenerates, moisturizes, and heals the skin

PATCHOULI

Botanical name: *Pogostemon Patchouli* or
Pogostemon Cablin
Scent: Musty
Patchouli grows to about three feet and has
whorls of light-purple or lavender flowers.

EFFECTS ON THE MIND AND EMOTIONS
mood uplifting
aphrodisiac
euphoric
nerve stimulant
interferes with sleep

EFFECT ON THE BODY
healing to the skin

OTHER USES
repels insects

PEPPER (BLACK)

Botanical name: *Piper Nigrum*
Scent: Hot and spicy
Black pepper is a tropical climbing vine that
grows to a height of about 10 feet and has
clusters of small white flowers.

EFFECTS ON THE MIND AND EMOTIONS
improves mental clarity and memory
reviving
stimulating

EFFECTS ON THE BODY
warming
loosens tight muscles
improves digestion in small amounts
improves the benefits of other oils when combined

Precaution: Essential oil of black pepper can irritate the skin.

PEPPERMINT

Botanical name: *Mentha Piperita*
Scent: Strong mint
Peppermint is a cross between mints and has been known since the 17th century. It grows to a height of one to three feet and has a purplish stem and pale violet flowers.

EFFECTS ON THE MIND AND EMOTIONS
mood uplifting
helps relieve mental fatigue
improves mental clarity, alertness, concentration, and memory
sharpens the senses
refreshing
reviving
energizing
nerve stimulant
aphrodisiac
encourages communication

EFFECTS ON THE BODY
cooling
relieves pain
increases physical strength and endurance
reduces inflammation
the vapors help breathing
improves digestion
increases the appetite
reduces lactation in nursing mothers
soothes itching skin

OTHER USES
disinfectant
repels insects

PERU BALSAM

Botanical name: *Myroxylon Pereirae*
Scent: Vanilla
Peru balsam is a slow-growing evergreen that grows to 60–120 feet and has fragrant flowers.

EFFECTS ON THE MIND AND EMOTIONS
calming
mood uplifting
promotes restful sleep
reduces stress
helpful for meditation

EFFECTS ON THE BODY
warming
loosens tight muscles
purifying
healing to the skin

OTHER USES
fixative for fragrances

PETITGRAIN

Botanical name: *Citrus Biguarade*
Scent: Sweet floral, citrus
Petitgrain is produced from the twigs and leaves of the orange, lemon, or tangerine tree.

EFFECTS ON THE MIND AND EMOTIONS
calming
mood uplifting

promotes restful sleep
reduces anxiety, tension, and stress
improves mental clarity, alertness, and memory
helpful for meditation

EFFECTS ON THE BODY
cooling
healing to the skin

PINE

Botanical name: *Pinus Sylvestris*
Scent: Fresh pine
Pine is an evergreen tree that grows to a height of 115–130 feet and has greenish-blue needle-like leaves. There are 90 species in the pine family. It is estimated pine trees can live for 1200 years.

EFFECTS ON THE MIND AND EMOTIONS
mood uplifting
helps relieve mental fatigue
improves mental clarity, alertness, and memory
refreshing
reviving

EFFECTS ON THE BODY
lessens pain
the vapors help breathing
helps in the reduction of cellulite deposits
purifying

OTHER USES
disinfectant

ROSE

Botanical name: *Rosa Centifolia* or *Rosa Damascena*
Scent: Sweet floral
The rose bush grows to various heights and produces sweet fragrant flowers.

EFFECTS ON THE MIND AND EMOTIONS
calming
mood uplifting
reduces stress
aphrodisiac

EFFECTS ON THE BODY
cooling
lessens aches and pains
reduces inflammation
balances the female hormonal and reproductive system
purifying
healing to the skin

ROSEMARY

Botanical name: *Rosmarinus Officinalis*
Scent: Fresh camphor-like
Rosemary is an evergreen shrub growing to two to six feet with needle-shaped leaves and blue flowers. The entire plant is aromatic.

EFFECTS ON THE MIND AND EMOTIONS
mood uplifting
helps relieve mental fatigue
improves mental clarity, alertness, and memory
sharpens the senses
refreshing
nerve stimulant

EFFECTS ON THE BODY
warming
relaxes tight muscles
relieves aches and pains
the vapors help breathing
improves digestion
helps in the reduction of cellulite deposits
purifying

OTHER USES
disinfectant
repels insects

SAGE (SPANISH)

Botanical name: *Salvia Lavendulafolia*
Scent: Spicy
Sage is an evergreen plant that grows to a height of two to three feet and has small light-blue to purple flowers and aromatic greyish-green leaves. There are about 500 different varieties of sage.

EFFECTS ON THE MIND AND EMOTIONS
improves mental clarity and alertness
reduces stress

EFFECTS ON THE BODY
relaxes tight muscles
lessens aches and pains
improves digestion
reduces lactation in nursing mothers
reduces perspiration
helps in the reduction of cellulite
purifying

OTHER USES
disinfectant

Precaution: Some of the varieties of sage contain the toxic component of thujone. Essential oil of Spanish sage is relatively non-toxic.

SANDALWOOD

Botanical name: *Santalum Album*
Scent: Woody
Sandalwood is an evergreen tree that grows to a height of 30 feet and has small purple flowers and small fruits containing a seed. There are 10 species of sandalwood.

EFFECTS ON THE MIND AND EMOTIONS
calming
mood uplifting
promotes restful sleep
reduces stress
aphrodisiac
encourages communication
brings out emotions
helpful for meditation

EFFECTS ON THE BODY
healing to the skin

OTHER USES
fixative for fragrances

SEA BUCKTHORN

Botanical name: *Hippophae Rhamnoides*
Scent: Sweet fruity
Sea buckthorn is a shrub that grows to a height of about 30 feet and has clusters of yellow flowers that develop into small orange berries.

EFFECTS ON THE MIND AND EMOTIONS
relaxing
mood uplifting

EFFECTS ON THE BODY
warming
loosens tight muscles
softens the skin
Note: Sea buckthorn is considered a vegetal/carrier oil, not an essential oil, and has valuable properties similar to essential oils.

SPEARMINT

Botanical name: *Mentha Spicata*
Scent: Minty
Spearmint grows to a height of one to three feet and has small white or lilac flowers and shiny green leaves.

EFFECTS ON THE MIND AND EMOTIONS
mood uplifting
helps relieve mental fatigue
improves mental clarity, alertness, and memory
sharpens the senses
refreshing
reviving
energizing
nerve stimulant
aphrodisiac
encourages communication

EFFECTS ON THE BODY
cooling
relieves aches and pains
increases physical strength and endurance
reduces inflammation
the vapors help breathing

improves digestion
increases the appetite
soothes itching skin

OTHER USES
repels insects

SPIKENARD

Botanical name: *Nardostachys Jatamansi*
Scent: Sweet woody
Spikenard is an aromatic plant that grows to a height of about two feet.

EFFECTS ON THE MIND AND EMOTIONS
calming
mood uplifting
promotes restful sleep
reduces stress

EFFECTS ON THE BODY
reduces inflammation

SPRUCE

Botanical name: *Picea Mariana*
Scent: Sweet pine-like
Spruce is an evergreen tree that grows to a height of 70–200 feet. There are about 50 species in the spruce family. It is estimated the tree can live for 1200 years.

EFFECTS ON THE MIND AND EMOTIONS
calming
mood uplifting
improves mental clarity
encourages communication
brings out feelings

EFFECTS ON THE BODY
breaks up congestion
the vapors help breathing

OTHER USES
disinfectant

TANGERINE

Botanical name: *Citrus Reticulata*
Scent: Sweet citrus
Tangerine is an evergreen citrus tree that
grows to about 20 feet and has fragrant
white flowers that develop into edible fruits.

EFFECTS ON THE MIND AND EMOTIONS
calming
mood uplifting
promotes restful sleep
relieves stress and tension
improves mental clarity and alertness
sharpens the senses

EFFECTS ON THE BODY
cooling
helps in the reduction of cellulite deposits
purifying
Precaution: Essential oil of tangerine can irritate dry skin. Skin can burn if exposed to
sunlight after topical application.

TEA TREE

Botanical name: *Melaleuca Alternifolia*
Scent: Camphor-like
Tea tree is an evergreen growing to 10 feet. It has
needle-like leaves and purple or yellow flowers;
belongs to a family of over 150 species of trees.

EFFECTS ON THE MIND AND EMOTIONS
mood uplifting
improves mental clarity
reviving
stimulating

EFFECTS ON THE BODY
relieves pain
the vapors help breathing
healing to the skin

OTHER USES
disinfectant
soothes the skin after insect bites

THYME

Botanical name: *Thymus Vulgaris*
Scent: Hot and spicy
Thyme is an evergreen plant that grows to
one foot and has small leaves and pink or
pale lilac flowers.

EFFECTS ON THE MIND AND EMOTIONS
mood uplifting
improves mental clarity, alertness, and memory
sharpens the senses
stimulating
relaxes the nerves

EFFECTS ON THE BODY
warming
relaxes tight muscles
relieves aches and pains
increases physical strength and energy
breaks up congestion
reduces inflammation
the vapors help breathing

improves digestion
promotes perspiration
helps in the reduction of cellulite deposits
purifying

OTHER USES
disinfectant
repels insects
Precaution: Essential oil of thyme can irritate
the skin.

VANILLA

Botanical name: *Vanilla Planifolia*
Scent: Sweet vanilla
Vanilla is a climbing plant that grows to
about 12 feet with clusters of flowers.

EFFECTS ON THE MIND AND EMOTIONS
calming
promotes restful sleep
mood uplifting
reduces stress
aphrodisiac
Note: Vanilla extracted by the CO_2 method is
recommended for use in the formulas.

VETIVER

Botanical name: *Vetiveria Zizanoides*
Scent: Earthy
Vetiver is a grass that grows to a height of four
to eight feet.

EFFECTS ON THE MIND AND EMOTIONS
calming
mood uplifting

promotes restful sleep
removes stress and tension

EFFECTS ON THE BODY
relaxes tight muscles
relieves pain
improves digestion
healing to the skin

OTHER USES
repels insects

YLANG-YLANG

Botanical name: *Cananga Odorata*
Scent: Sweet floral
Ylang-Ylang is an evergreen tree that grows
to a height of about 100 feet and has large,
fragrant yellow flowers and glossy leaves.

EFFECTS ON THE MIND AND EMOTIONS
calming
mood uplifting
promotes restful sleep
reduces stress
aphrodisiac
euphoric
encourages communication
brings out feelings

EFFECTS ON THE BODY
relaxes tight muscles
lessens pain

OTHER USES
disinfectant

About the Authors

David Schiller and Carol Schiller have been blending aromatherapy formulations since 1986 and instructing aromatherapy classes for colleges and other educational organizations since 1989. They are the authors of *500 Formulas for Aromatherapy* (Sterling) and numerous magazine articles on the subject of aromatherapy.

Carol Schiller is also a certified hypnotherapist and graphologist and has instructed classes on these subjects as well.

INDEX

itch relief powders, 67–68

itch relief, 8

Juniper Berry, *Juniperus Communis,* 114

lavender, *Lavandula Officinalis* or *Lavandula Augustifolia,* 114–115

lemon, *Citrus Limonum,* 115

lemongrass, *Cymbopogon Citratus,* 115–116

life length, plants, *See* Cypress; Pine; Spruce

light bulb rings, 14

lime, *Citrus Limetta,* 116

lips, chapped, 64–65

litsea cubeba, *Litsea Cubeba,* 116

lovers, for, 59–60

loving oneself, 23, 37–40

lunch menus, 100

mandarin, *Citrus Nobilis,* 116–117

marjoram, *Origanum Majorana* or *Majorana Hortensis,* 117

massage, 15, 31, 57–58, 80, 83–84, 93–94

measurements, 18

medications, 18

meditation, 23–24, 40–42

mental concentration, 42–46

mind conditioning, 21
   power of, 19–56

mist sprays, 15, 26, 30, 32, 35–36, 39–40, 41–42, 45–46, 48, 50, 54, 77, 79, 81, 84–85, 85–86, 89–90, 96–97

mood uplifting, 60–61

motivation, 22, 46

mouthwash, 68–69

myrrh, *Commiphora Myrrha,* 117

myrtle, *Myrtus Communis,* 117–118

nature, 7-8

neroli, *Citrus Aurantium,* 118

nutmeg, *Myristica Fragrans,* 118

oils, essential
   dilute, 17
   definition, 13
   extraction, 13
   profiles, 103–125
   handling, 18
   pure, 17
   pure carrier, 17
   safety, 17–18

orange, *Citrus Aurantium* or *Citrus Sinensis,* 118

oregano, *Origanum Vulgare,* 118–119

palmarosa, *Cymbopogon Martini,* 119

patchouli, *Pogostemon Patchouli* or *Pogostemon Cablin,* 119

pepper (black), *Piper Nigrum,* 119–120

peppermint, *Menta Piperita,* 120

Peru balsam, *Myroxylon Pereirae,* 120

petitgrain, *Citrus Biguarada,* 120–121

pili nuts. *See* Elemi

pine, *Pinus Sylvestris,* 121

plants and aromas 10-11

powders
   body, 14
   itch relief, 67
   shave, 69–70

pregnancy, 17

reflection, 22, 48–51
   worksheet, 51

refreshing, 59

relaxation, 24

relaxing, 61–62

rosemary, *Rosmarinus Officinalis,* 121–122

rose, *Rosa Centifolia* or *Rosa Damascena,* 121

sage (Spanish), *Salvia Lavendulafolia,* 122

sample menus, 99–101

sandalwood, *Santalum Album,* 122

sauna, facial, 66–67

sauna/steam room, 85–86

sauna/steam room, 15–16

sea buckthorn, *Hippophae Rhamnoides,* 122–123

sebum, 63

self-preservation, 8

shaping up, 91–101

skin, 17, 18, 63

sleep, 73, 78-79

snoring, 8
   stop, 79–81

spearmint, *Mentha Spicata,* 123

spikenard, *Nardostachys Jatamansi,* 123

spruce, *Picea Mariana,* 123–124

steam inhalation, 16

Stevenson, Robert Louis, 22

stress
   surrender your, 73–90
   reducers, 81–86

tangerine, *Citrus Reticulata,* 124

tea tree, *Melaleuca Alternifolia,* 124

thyme, *Thymus Vulgaris,* 124–125

touch
   growth: stimulates, impairs, 56
   need for, 57–62

tree, holy, 7

urban living benefits, 7

vanilla, *Vanilla Planifolia,* 125

vetiver, *Vetiveria Zizanoides,* 125

visualization, 21

Winters, Jason, 20

worksheets, 27, 30, 33, 36, 51, 55, 56

ylang-ylang, *Cananga Odorata,* 125

yoga, 8, 86–90

yogi, 19